A Sociological View of AIDS

This series, an academic masterpiece on AIDS research in the Chinese sociological community in the past two decades, analyzes in detail the situations of a range of people living with HIV/AIDS from various perspectives. By providing valuable theoretical insights and assessing counter measures, it not only allows readers to gain a thorough understanding of AIDS-related social realities, promotes the interpretation and implementation of social policies and the role of sociology in AIDS prevention and treatment, but also helps to coordinate the interests and needs of all party involved in order to handle relations between different groups of people and promote the formulation and adjustment of relevant policies, laws and regulations.

More information about this series at https://link.springer.com/bookseries/16458

Suiming Pan

The Social Construction of AIDS Issues

華中科技大學出版社
Huazhong University of Science and Technology Press

Springer

Suiming Pan
Beijing, China

Translated by
Hulin Zhao
Jiangsu University of Technology
Changzhou, China

ISSN 2662-5954 ISSN 2662-5962 (electronic)
A Sociological View of AIDS
ISBN 978-981-16-7518-8 ISBN 978-981-16-7519-5 (eBook)
https://doi.org/10.1007/978-981-16-7519-5

Jointly published with Huazhong University of Science and Technology Press
The print edition is not for sale in China (Mainland). Customers from China (Mainland) please order the print book from: Huazhong University of Science and Technology Press.

Translation from the *Chinese Simplified* language edition: *艾滋病问题的社会重构* by Suiming Pan,

This Springer imprint is published by the registered company Springer Nature Singapore Pte Ltd.
The registered company address is: 152 Beach Road, #21-01/04 Gateway East, Singapore 189721, Singapore

Contents

Chapter 1
The Social Construction of AIDS Issue and Its Significance

Making an overall analysis of a country or society as a whole has always been the unique strength of sociological studies. However, the necessity of Sociology of AIDS does not originate from this alone, but that AIDS has been recognized as not only a medical problem, also a social difficulty worldwide since the 1920s.

But why? Why had AIDS became a social issue while there are a variety of intractable diseases more serious than it? Why do HIV patients can enjoy such a decent social welfare policy as "Four Frees and One Care". Obviously, we can't make it clear with medical or public health theory. Then, I might as well embark on a book writing based on this fundamental question.

1.1 Why AIDS Becomes an "Issue"?

Since the first report of the AIDS patient in 1985, the epidemic of AIDS in China can be roughly divided into three major phases: emerging of imported cases (1985–1988), local spreading stage (1989–1993) and high-speed growth period (1994–now). What's worse, it has spread from high-risk groups to general population relentlessly.

Nowadays, in China, the highly moralized AIDS is no longer a traditional disease in biological field. Instead, it is a "problem" which has been put many labels on by our society. A consensus is emerging in Chinese society: it is imperative to develop the traditional treatment methods on AIDs, which are now confined to medical and biological modes, into overall strategic system with the guidance of social sciences, arts and humanities.

At present, most of the AIDS research in China is still limited to the hygienic field and operational level. Biomedical and epidemiological terms have become the dominant discourse in AIDS research. Several sociological research about AIDS mainly focuses on different sides and solutions of it. Although such research have added new social and cultural information to the issue of AIDS, or in turn, reflected the sociological research from the perspective of AIDS, the concept of "AIDS"

S. Pan, *The Social Construction of AIDS Issues*, A Sociological View of AIDS,
https://doi.org/10.1007/978-981-16-7519-5_1

and its underlying significance have not yet obtained enough concerns in China. Besides, there is also a lack of questioning and deconstruction of the dominating AIDS discourse.

In Europe and America, it's emerging and being increasingly valued to make a historical and procedural analysis of established social concepts like homosexuality, heterosexuality and sexuality from the perspective of social construction. At the same time, I believe that the possible solution to AIDS as a social issue lies with the construction ways, mechanism and process of it in the current China.

Then, which type of AIDS and the conflicting conceptions does China have? Why AIDS has become a tough issue? What a problem it is? Why it is such like? What's the logic behind it? If we do not make such problems clear, the likelihood of finding the best way to solve the problems will be greatly reduced, whether in the theoretical level or practical level.

The basic streamline of this chapter is: analyzing the AIDS from a relatively macro perspective rather than concrete operational methods, and making the construction of AIDS instead of its transmission level in the context of China as the main line. Firstly, I begin with the theoretical analysis and its social significance, which is different from simple conflicts between different schools. Secondly, I analyze the contest of various social power in the process of AIDS being constructed and concluded, rather than making different explanation of policies. Last but not least, I elaborate on the central proposition, i.e., the "AIDS issue" is a symbol of China's social restructuring process. And only in an effort to advance such process can we be more likely to find the best problem-solving mode (rather than clamoring repeatedly or giving countermeasures alone).

1.1.1 Conflicting Conceptions on AIDS and Its Social and Cultural Significance

(1) **Conflicting conceptions on AIDS**

① The argument between behavior science, social sciences, and arts and humanities

The two sides focus on whether AIDS is an individual or socio-cultural behavior. At the very beginning, most people constructed AIDS issue from a medical perspective only, and tended to deal with the disease on its merits. With the deepening practices of AIDS prevention and control, more and more people with this opinion began to pay heed to behavioral issues, such as the situation of condom use, and the reason why people do not want to use condoms and so on. It is undeniable that we have made considerable important results by doing so.

The internal logic of this construction is that behavior happens to the individual and is mainly determined by the individual himself. The most prominent manifestation is the "KABP" questionnaire and research methods, which was introduced to China by the World Health Organization (WTO) and other international organizations at the latest 1990. The basic hypothesis of "KABP" is that one's practice (P) depends on the combination of his knowledge (K), attitude (A) and belief (B).

This kind of thinking mode based on simple linear deduction, along with the help of the continuous hard indoctrination by powerful international organizations, occupies the prime position in the practices of AIDS prevention in China. It demonstrates the absolute preponderance of cognitive psychology in this field.

On the contrary, social sciences, arts and humanities emphasize that only when human behavior interacts with the specific situation in a specific social culture, can it jointly form an observable manifestation of practice with certain social and cultural interpretation and significance. If this aspect is ignored, our understanding of human behavior will suffer a great loss both in depth and breadth, and the possibility of misunderstanding "high-risk behavior" and ineffective AIDS prevention efforts will increase dramatically.

For example, it is difficult to understand the rate of condom use among female sex workers with KABP method alone. They live in a society with gender inequality materialized by whoremaster; their political and economic rights have been deprived with high share of income plundered by their various higher-ups; they have been stigmatized because of the extreme lack of support system and information sources; they are traditionalized since they care more about their fertility than infection of HIV/AIDS, and more the risk of being arrested than contracting AIDS. Their practices are, in fact, the production of making a living in specific situation. The risk of contracting AIDS is only annexed into this interaction as a cost. Therefore, if the prevention and treatment of AIDS do not consider other factors, but merely inculcate prevention knowledge, it will be very difficult for them to make further prevention practice (P), and even more difficult to achieve the goal of "100% condom use", no matter how much knowledge (K) they have, how correct their attitudes (A) are, and how firm their beliefs (B) are.

Furthermore, KABP has greater potential to lead our work to fragmentation. KABP method, for example, does little to explain the stagnation in condom use among female sex workers when the usage rate has risen to a certain level in areas where HIV/AIDS prevention has been well established.

On the contrary, social sciences, arts and humanities find and emphasize that the organizational form of the "sex industry" and its development specificity play a huge role in the behaviors of all individuals. It is advocated to view and solve problems from the perspective of the four categories of "sex industry", which mainly involves the mutual relations and interactions between stakeholders.

② The hegemony of economics and the weak social sciences, arts and humanities

With regard to this, the debate focuses on "what are the socio-economic impacts of AIDS? And how deep the impacts are?". To some extent, such debates have given rise to a academic war. In general, the economic construction, which tends to use quantitative data to calculate the harm of AIDS spreading on economic development, has become the mainstream discourse, at least in China currently.

However, the emphasis of the construction from the perspective of social sciences, arts and humanities mainly falls on what and how AIDS and AIDS prevention and treatment affect community reconstruction, social development and human development.

These two perspectives seem perfectly compatible with each other in a purely speculative manner. But in the specific practice of prevention and treatment of AIDS, they lead to different technical routes, and thus achieve very different results. For example, a program to fight AIDS in a town. It follows the path of economic construction, basically solving the problem of local employment of HIV-infected people, that is, it avoids the negative impact of labor loss on economic development. However, as this solution mainly relies on the project funds to start and continue, the infected people have not formed their own organizational strength, nor have the ability to coordinate and negotiate with the local administrative system. As a result, their independently sustainable development ability is not ideal, and the possibility of large-scale promotion and application still remains uncertain. In addition, in the social environment where a large number of rural labor have to go to cities for work, the practical effect of this "local employment" solution model also needs further discussing. Conversely, if the project made community building and social organization building as its main goals, it would be more likely to succeed.

(2) **The social significance of conflicting conceptions on AIDS**

This conflict actually reflects the contradiction and struggle between different social forces. The following is my analysis of its basic notion, value orientation and specific operation respectively.

① **Basic Notion**

A typical expression of the basic notion is: if the AIDS epidemic spreads in a large scale, the consequences will be "the destruction of the achievements of reform and opening up", "the destructive impact on economic development", "the reduction of the number of labor force", and "the decrease of GDP", and so on. The implied logic is that man is merely a material producer, so we should evaluate his value and life and death with economic indicators.

Another notion emphasizes that the fight against AIDS is primarily for "safeguarding the individual's right to keep healthy", "the right to health being a fundamental human right", and "embodying equity in health care", as such. The internal logic is that human beings are the masters of the society first, so the realization of human rights is the fundamental indicator to evaluate the effectiveness of AIDS prevention and treatment work and the process of social development.

The conflict between these two basic notions is most evident in the question of estimating the extent of the current HIV/AIDS epidemic in China.

For the former one, the exaggeration of the prevalence of HIV/AIDS and the use of "scare tactics" can easily become an involuntary choice. In particular, it is easy to adopt the strategy of positioning AIDS as the enemy of economic development to attract the attention of higher authorities.

On the contrary, the latter tends to believe that the goal of the fight against AIDS is not only to control the increase in the number of people infected with AIDS, but also to promote the realization of the human health right. Therefore, it is not advisable to exaggerate the epidemic.

② **Value orientation**

The first value orientation was mainly reflected in the period from 1980 to 1990 when AIDS just became an "issue". During this period, AIDS was regard as "a fly from the outside China", and the infection of AIDS was regarded as "a deserved punishment of morally bad personnel". Moreover, some people even hold that "AIDS is good for racial cleansing". A similar moral orientation is the so-called "AbCism", which is short for abstinence (A) firstly, then being faithful to partners (B), and the last resort is to use condom (C). Find further Chinese expression about it on *AIDS ABC* written by Lauren Clark from America. It tends to use AIDS as the last weapon of purging morality. This value orientation has been restrained by public publicity since the late 1990s, but it is still deeply rooted in the hearts and actions of many people. The logic is actually quite simple: "Bad people should be at fault".

By the late 1990s, AIDS prevention and treatment efforts had increasingly reached the stage of intervention for "high-risk groups". Then the former logic is transformed to "majority at fault". The main idea is that all policies are designed to protect the majority, so the "high-risk groups" like whoremasters, prostitutes and drug addicts should not be rescued, instead, we should intensify efforts to eradicate them. This notion is the main reason for the awkward situation in which one executive branch cracks down and another one rescues in practice.

This logical fallacy has been proved in practice. As AIDS has spread from high-risk groups to the general population, the number of the so-called "bad guys" increased markedly, bringing disaster to more and more "good people" who meet the moral standards.

The second value orientation holds that AIDS is just a kind of disease, and HIV-infected people are just patients. Therefore, the fight against AIDS must combat any form of discrimination against those infected. The logic is simple: all men are created equal.

③ **Specific Operation**

The first tends to believe that human beings can overcome all obstacles with the help of advanced science and technology, since AIDS vaccine will be developed and popularized eventually, maybe in the near future. Its logic is: AIDS is a disease, so the final ways to defeat it can only rely on medicine. The rest of measures are only auxiliary means.

Another trend is that prevention is above everything else, so we have no time to bide for a vaccine and we should not have any expectation. Its logic is: since there are still no healed cases yet, we can only strive for fewer deaths.

Literally, the two ideas seem to go hand in hand. But for any large-scale AIDS prevention effort, there is a problem: how to allocate limited resources. People who hold these two views tend to think that the input and output of the other side are less than satisfactory.

Implicit in this conflict is a logical struggle: is man primarily an objective being governed (cured) by science and technology, or is he a subject capable of actively changing his destiny through choice?

Although neither of the two sides of the conflict would go to such an extreme and thus completely negate the value of the other's work, the struggle between the two logics is actually reflected in the concrete operation anytime and anywhere. After the successful practice of "cocktail therapy" in AIDS (A mixture of drugs used to treat a particular condition; while any mixture may be considered a 'cocktail'—e.g., antibiotics or chemotherapeutics—the term has had most currency in immunology as a mixture of immunosuppressive agents for controlling rejection), studies have found a decline in condom use, at least among certain "high-risk groups" in some places. In the interpretation of this phenomenon, advances in treatment will replace prevention and drugs weaken the argument for prevention. It is in fact an important aspect of the conflict between the two aforementioned logics in this chapter.

1.1.2 The Game Behind the "Highest Political Positioning"

Since the 1990s, the reported and measured number of AIDS in China has increased. By the latest 2001, some scholar's proposals and official's speeches can be seen on newspapers, such as: the AIDS epidemic is neither an epidemic issue nor a prophylactic one, but it is a social issue. On March 2004, the State Council's document finally made such a qualitative conclusion: "AIDS prevention and treatment is essential to economic development, social stability, national security and prosperity."

By December 2004, the document of China's Ministry of Public Health has once again interpreted it as: "AIDS prevention and treatment work is a major event concerning the quality of the nation and the rise and fall of the country". AIDS prevention must be "regarded as a strategic task of overall concern" and " a concrete manifestation of China's high responsibility for the survival and development of the international community and human beings".

This "highest political positioning" indicates that the construction of AIDS problem by the mainstream society in China has finally been established by the authority of the highest administration and the highest political mode. It links AIDS to almost all the most basic values and the highest ideals of China, which amounts to treating AIDS as "a matter of life and death" for China. At least this has formed a new "state policy" at the level of the concept.

Such definition is unprecedented in China for any disease, and it is also unique for almost all medical and health work since the founding of the People's Republic of China in1949.

I don't want to discuss such a qualitative conclusion, but to explore what social forces, considerations and strategies are used to ultimately build AIDS into such "a matter of life and death". It is hoped to explore the possibility of solving this problem.

(1) The politicization and international politicization of AIDS

Before the mid-1990s, AIDS, once seen as "a fly from the West", was cracked down on to "keep it out of the country". In other words, AIDS in China was politicized internationally for the first time under the guise of "international class struggle".

The second international politicization began at the latest mid-1990s. At that time, various international organizations started to intervene in the prevention and treatment of AIDS in China. Although many of them were to support China's health authorities for specific work to the prevention and treatment of HIV/AIDS, they were necessarily involved in China's domestic politics. That is "policy development", namely "strengthening strategic planning and management ability of the main public sector, and making more effective policy and strategy to control AIDS".

Such "policy development" inevitably involves not only the orientation or even some specific details of Chinese governments at all levels in the field of public health policy making, but also the government's allocation of financial strength and public resources to a certain extent, and even legislation, law enforcement and justice in some fields.

In the face of such foreign intervention, Chinese leaders at all levels have almost no unified and clear strategy for a long period of time, nor have they shown a clear response. Locally, this practice has yielded significant results, producing a series of planning and government regulatory documents. Some "concepts" have been "embedded" and have changed Chinese policy step by step.

Until December 1999, James D Wolfensohn, the then world bank president, specially wrote to President Jiang Zemin, and pointed out that AIDS was not only a health issue, but exerted the huge pressure on the entire public finance system. He was active to cooperate with the Chinese government, and willing to have the task of control AIDS on the Chinese policy agenda. In his reply, Jiang also pointed out the huge impact of the AIDS epidemic on families, communities and the whole society. Leaders at the highest levels of the country began to identify AIDS as a social issue and to pay some attention to it. Since then, the Chinese government had endorsed the UN's "Millennium Goals" (the sixth goal of it is to fight AIDS, tuberculosis and malaria), though it is not quite the same with the released tenth Five-Year Plan.

It was a symbolic turning point, I should say. It means that China is beginning to recognize the fact that AIDS is no longer an "internal affair" that cannot be interfered with by foreigners, and that all it needs to do is start "integrating with the world". What is most significant is that this huge and significant external push has come not from a professional body like the World Health Organization, nor even from international public opinion, but from the World Bank.

The practical effect of this turn is marketable. One is that China has begun to accept the international argument that "AIDS harms economic development" and derived a frightening "GDP loss rate" from the case of some African countries. It was not until 2004 that a political judgment at the heart of the country made, "AIDS was a matter of life and death".

In short, political forces at home and abroad move from confrontation to cooperation, strengthening and accelerating China's mainstream construction of AIDS as an issue. It finally presents a "passive globalization", albeit in the form of such strong emotion expressions as "national security" and "the rise and fall of the nation". Corresponding to the two international politicizations, AIDS has also been twice politicized in China.

The first one was the "class struggle" in the early stages of the AIDS epidemic (corresponding to the end of the Cold War in international politics); the second was the establishment of the "highest political position" in 2004, i.e., "a matter of life and death" (corresponding to the rise of "globalization"). The close correlation between these two politicized events at home and abroad reflects the leading role played by domestic political changes. The purpose of this chapter is not to discuss whether this statement is true or not, but to explore the structure and operation mechanism of the social forces that contribute to this statement.

(2) **The social power behind politicized AIDS**

① **The role of dedicated institutions**

In the middle 1990s when AIDS entered a rapidly growth period, the dedicated AIDS institutions began to emphasize the issue of leaders' insufficient concerns on AIDS for their own sake and the support of "policy development".

However, such changes of function make it more difficult and negligent for dedicated institutions to carry out original thinking. Thus the phenomenon of "path dependence" appears. That is, we may have to copy partially or even absolutely all the ideas, thinking and methods from all over the world in an effort to prove that the leaders' do not attach importance to it; we may struggle to raise AIDS to a new political height, still for the same reason. Consequently, it becomes the main domestic social force that directly advances the second politicization. Furthermore, thanks to the convention of drafting right, some officials working at the lower-level can participate in the decision making process of senior officials by drawing up relevant documents. But once the highest political position is established, the aforementioned force will be trapped in two awkward situations.

The first embarrassment comes from its self-preservation strategies: the extent of exploited capabilities of country's top leaders does not commensurate with the extent to which this force itself bears all responsibilities for the continued spread of the epidemic. The second comes from its path-dependent tendency. The need to fight AIDS according to the international value of human rights raises more than just decentralization of power and transfer of profit but the self-revolution.

As a result, although we never doubt the initiative and capabilities of medical workers in response to the AIDS, yet we still need to pay close attention to the development of dedicated institutions as a whole.

② **Feedback of the local authorities**

The AIDS-related local governmental departments ever showed manifestly negative and even resistant attitudes towards AIDS prevention and control for a long time. The key point is that their position of preventing and controlling AIDS is quite different from that of national dedicated institutions and the central government in their own benefit balancing. As such situation was constantly delivered to top central government, as well as repeatedly mentioned by international society, the central government finally raised the issue to the highest level of fundamental political tasks in its previous operation route. Along with sharp increase of direct government fund can local authorities be pushed to make a difference in this field.

However, around the twenty-first century, the strong financial support from international society has prompted local governments to see AIDS from the perspective of finance, and shift their attitudes in a more positive manner. As a result, many breakthrough policy developments began to take the path of local origin and then feedback to the central government, advancing the concept of "highest political position".

③ The promotion of perceived public needs

Under the effect of "SARS" crisis, the general Chinese people have increased their public health demands markedly. Naturally, treating AIDS has been compared, thought about and involved into the top public health demand What's more, this demand was finally being perceived both by the people themselves and by the government. All these lay the basic foundation for public opinion and historical timing for the construction of AIDS as "a matter of life and death".

④ The secondary attack of sexual culture

In China, the onset of the AIDS epidemic coincided with the debut and increasingly fierce "sexual revolution". No matter what attitude people hold to it, they have to bear the impact of this historical change.

The close correlation between AIDS and sex is an important reason why society highly values it. Besides, for the past several years, there some people have always disregarded the fact that HIV was mostly transmitted by blood rather than the sexual transmission. It strengthened the "sensibility" of AIDS and somehow fostered the politicalized AIDS.

⑤ Supportive factors from the emerging medium power

The spread of AIDS in China keeps in line with the secularized media development on the whole. No matter what attitudes the mass media has, it has continuously contributed to the politicized problem of AIDS, one of the most attracting fodders. It's true that the conditions and voice of people who are actually related to AIDS have been delivered because of various media power.

⑥ Push from the idea of non-governmental organizations

The concept of non-governmental organization and its ideas may not originate from but significantly developed due to the AIDS issue.

According to the current international standards, China's large-scale non-governmental organizations are still in rudiment, but as an ideal and a feasible possibility, it indicates the fact that government will meet its antagonist in settling the issue of AIDS. It is hard to predict, but the non-governmental organizations do play an urging role for the fact that "highest political positioning" occupies the moral high ground.

⑦ The Convenience of Absence of Vital Stakeholders

Beyond doubt, the HIV-infected patients and those living with them are the main stakeholders of AIDS, at least in China. Nevertheless, such people have little opportunity to express their claims, let alone fight for the protection of their rights and interests. However, this absence removes possible interference and additional considerations for the positioning of mainstream construction. Thus making it easier to apply such non-individualized concepts as "economic development, society stability, national security and rise and fall of nation".

⑧ The Present Political Background: The Urgent Need of Populist Policy

The slogan of "building a harmonious society" reflects the fact that Chinese government has conducted a series of policies close to common people. Under the joint efforts of the aforementioned forces, as well as out of the strategic consideration of highest political enforcement, the central government began to make AIDS prevention and control as a starting point and demonstration of its new policy, and adopted many unprecedented forceful measures, thus laying the core power of constructing the matter of life and death. According to the original interpretation of the Ministry of Health: it is the embodiment of practicing important thought of "three represents" and "building the party that serves the public and governs for the people", and it is the concrete embodiment of adhering to the people-oriented principle and implementing the scientific outlook on development. So from these facts, we can see that social governors have realized that the good conduct of AIDS prevention and control will benefit mass people and bring huge social benefit to themselves too.

⑨ The Third Time of AIDS Being Politicized: Reconsideration of Mainstream Construction Positioning

The "highest political positioning" of the AIDS issue in 2004 did not bring an end to thinking, but provided a higher starting point for the third attempt to make it politicized internationally.

This can be attributed more or less to the aforementioned "economic loss-oriented" approach. This orientation leads to a wishful logic: since China has put AIDS at a political height that is related to economic development, social stability, national security and prosperity, then power from international level will no longer criticize us and we will be on an equal footing with them. But in fact, this is an incomprehension and underestimation to the international "AIDS politics". The most important change brought by the transition of "highest political positioning" to China is that the specific content of "connecting with international standards" can hardly be controlled well. As a result, international concepts which were previously considered as incompatible with China's national conditions began to enter China on a large scale,. Besides, a kind of constructing force based on social equity and human rights also emerged in China. A growing number of Chinese scholars changed their focus of this issue. They began to emphasize the health hazards of AIDS to the right to health, which is one of the basic human rights, and to stress that the prevention and treatment of

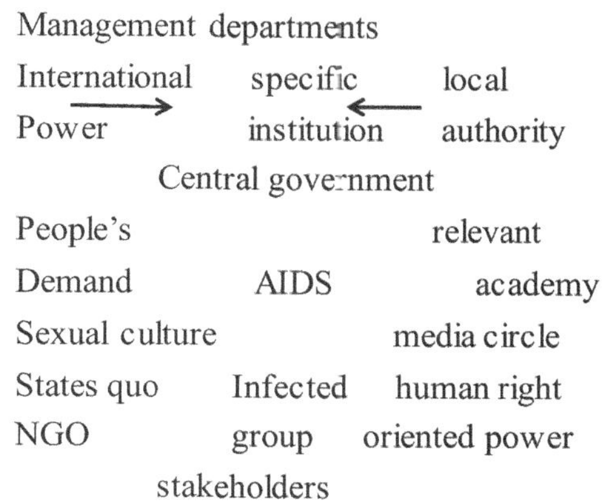

Fig. 1.1 Management departments

AIDS is a matter of overall human rights situation of a society as a whole, instead of merely highlighting the protection of the infected people's personal rights.

Accordingly, the right to health, reform of the system of social justice and health, the social vulnerable groups, gender equality, the role of non-governmental organizations, and public intellectuals and public space, democratic policies together, of which seems to has nothing to do with AIDS, were all put forward, discussed recently in the field of AIDS prevention. So much so that it has became a public opinion to some extent.

Behind the third international politicization lies the conflict between the international mainstream forces and China's national interests. That is, whether the prevention and treatment of AIDS should be regarded as a powerful means to promote human rights and social equity. From such a perspective, although the third politicization of AIDS in international arena hasn't became the mainstream of China, its appearance shows some changes in China's national interests and national orientation. From the various phenomena described above, we can draw a picture of why AIDS is framed as a social issue (Fig. 1.1).

From the above diagram, we can get triple meanings.

Firstly, The country's fundamental political decisions on "AIDS being a matter of life and death" are driven less by political wisdom at the highest level than by a combination of "international forces", "competent authorities" and "local power". Many scholars have discussed the problems of management system reflected in it.

Secondly, although the central government remains the main constructor, resource provider and policy maker of "AIDS issue" in terms of strength, it is no longer at the top of the pyramid in terms of structure. It is now in an approximately circular multi-link. And from the perspective of operational mechanism, though the "national will" is still strong, we must connect it with the three forces of "society", "public opinion" and "vital stakeholders", forming a "concerted circle", if we want to put it into effect. This suggests that in today's China, the source, composition and direction of action of the highest political decisions, like "AIDS is a matter of life and death", have shown a tendency of diversification, and even began to be dispersed to a certain extent.

Thirdly, the "vital stakeholders" of AIDS such as the infected person and his/her life circle, have played little role in the construction of the AIDS issue so far. The "non-governmental organization" and "building forces of human rights orientation" are pretty much the same. This means that the "concerted circle" of the construction of "AIDS issue" and the implementation of AIDS prevention and treatment work is incomplete in real life. In this chapter, I think that this is the real social significance of "AIDS issue".

1.1.3 "AIDS Issue": A Symbol of Social Restructuring in China

As we all know, the above situation is by no means unique to the AIDS field. It deeply shows that not AIDS as an issue has been politicized, but the overall structure and operation mechanism of Chinese society have been put a label like "AIDS" on a specific problem. The background and implication is that "Chinese society has entered an era of interests gaming", indicating that Chinese society needs a process of restructuring, which has already begun.

"Chinese social restructuring" refers to the recombination of various factors and people who constitute the society on the whole. And the value orientation is to form a new form of harmonious society. In this chapter, I will take it as a cut-and-dried concept to start a discussion. However, this chapter is not a monograph on this subject but some hypothetical propositions, which will not enjoy deep analysis. At the same time, social restructuring at least includes social management system, market system, public space and international interaction, but this chapter will focus on society in the narrow sense.

Social restructuring was put forward based on the judgment that the present Chinese society is not just a matter of class differentiation, it is the fragmentation of the whole social structure. Some scholars believe that the current social differentiation is a diversified and overlapping kind, which does not lead to well-defined social class, but some interest groups at most. These groups are like fragments, showing no signs of assembling into large stratum. As a result, they argue that the current social differentiation tends to be "fragmented". For example, in *The Stratification of Chinese Society during Transitional Period*, Li Qiang mentioned that the diversification of class interests is characterized by fragmentation, "loose sand" and even atomization; the social operation mechanism is characterized by "virtualization". It mainly refers to the fact that the operation of the society as a whole has fallen into a superficiality, show and aphasia. In other words, few people implement and evaluate the social operation seriously. Of course, this chapter merely provides a hypothetical measurement, but it doesn't mean that the current China is completely such like. These trends go in the same direction, so it is far more enough to harmonize the various aspects of the existing social structures. The current Chinese society is not really a matter of "transformation" from one model to another, but how to bring the various social components together again. It is precisely because that AIDS emerged in the process of social restructuring in China and had a huge impact on China's society, so that it become an "issue" in time, and a marker of social reconstruction. SARS disappeared too quickly and too soon to become a sign like AIDS. To this, this chapter has the following arguments.

(1) **The relationship between AIDS and social problems**

The current situation of the AIDS epidemic in China is mainly caused by various social factors, rather than the result of the "natural" transmission of HIV. The prevalence of AIDS is not a problem that only affects the society, but a problem that originates from the society, such as organizational mechanism, cultural background, social environment and thoughts and so on.

For example, "sex services" or the so-called "prostitution and whoring" is an important way to spread HIV.The conclusion of the former Ministry of Health, the current National Health Commission, was that "sexual transmission contact rate increased". However, neither "buying" nor "providing" sexual services is simply a matter of personal morality. When I led a research group to investigate AIDS transmission in a southwest town in the summer of 2002, I found the transmission mechanism below:

- Local governors want to build a development zone in such a poverty-stricken and remote rural area;
- So they bulldozed the two village land but only built two broad town highway;
- The houses on both sides of the road were all built by local farmers and residents with their land compensation or fund raising;
- However, no investors came here, so the phenomenon like "sellers are more than buyers" appeared;
- Then cultivating "street girls" became the only way to make a living, consequently the locals had to use these houses running the "entertainment places";
- Since there were very few customers, "street girls" constantly left here;
- Bosses had to go to the labor market in the nearby city to abduct more girls, and confine them;
- Here being the training base of "street girls";
- In such an environment, those "street girls" generally don't use condoms;
- As a result, venereal disease became very common in these "street girls", and constantly spread over a long distance when they fled.

In this "mechanism", it is not the venereal diseases first and then harm to the society, but social problems come first and then push the spread of venereal diseases.

Although the case studies mentioned above are not representative, it should be a realistic recognition that the three routes of AIDS transmission (blood transmission, sexual transmission and mother-to-child transmission) did not exist in China in the last 20 years from the perspective of historical development. This means that from a macro point of view, the whole AIDS issue in China is later than the emergence of some social problems.

One of the most typical examples is the fact that farmers in some regions are infected with AIDS by selling blood, which is a very rare case in the world. To date, despite the increase of drug and sexual transmission, the majority have been infected through blood sales linked to poverty or even local policies. It continues to demonstrate the fallacy of "natural transmission" and the clarity of the "social product" judgment.

(2) The risk of life and panic caused by AIDS

For the whole society, the harm of AIDS is not the disease itself, but the social panic it brings about. Although AIDS is a chronic infectious disease, it is endowed with too many moral meanings. Even some propagandas and educational work aimed at preventing AIDS unconsciously reinforce this moral meaning. This is where the "AIDS panic" appears, and the level of panic increases exponentially and is greater than it actually is. In early 2002, there was a rumor in Tianjin that people gave an injection to others with the blood of the infected. It not only caused the biggest social panic in Tianjin at that time, but also affected Beijing seriously.

The subsequent SARS epidemic demonstrated once again that such public health crises, including the high prevalence of AIDS, can be solved by existing social mechanisms if they are merely concerned with deaths and impacts on the economic development. But, in fact, it has caused widespread and profound panic in society. It is such fear, rather than the disease itself, that temporarily disrupts the functioning of whole societies in some places, even in capitals and metropolises. Its historical experience is that the process of social restructuring cannot cope with such sudden and widespread disasters. Accordingly, our government has intensified efforts in social restructuring to reduce the possibility of a recurrence of the disaster.

(3) The tendency of class selection in AIDS susceptible population

The harm of AIDS to Chinese society mainly lies not in how many but in what kind of people are infected. And we have to see this question in two different aspects.

In terms of blood transmission (blood selling and syringe-sharing when taking drugs) and mother-to-child transmission, AIDS victims are more socially disadvantaged, because their economic conditions and social status prevent them from taking relatively expensive precaution measures. In this sense, AIDS is actually a "disease of poverty", so the role of simple publicity and education is very limited. The problem needs to be completely solved through social restructuring. But in terms of sexual transmission, AIDS tends to be a "disease of affluence". In this chapter, I will start with the results of four surveys conducted in 2000, 2006, 2010 and 2015 respectively. Find details in the opening remarks of the third article in *Sexuality of the Chinese People during 2000–2015*.

The survey showed that male factory directors, managers and bosses were not only the most likely to engage in prostitution among all nine classes, but also ten times the urban male manual workers and various rural male laborers. They also had the most other sexual partners of any class, and as many times as workers and farmers.

Men in the top 5 percent of earners were also more likely to engage in prostitution dozens of times than those in the bottom 40 percent.

This survey indicates to a large extent that such current "economic elites" are far more likely to act as the "bridge population" for the spread of AIDS than the masses. Moreover, any existing force and measures in the current society can hardly restrict their sexual relations and the spread of AIDS brought by them. This is both a product of social problems and a proof of the necessity of social restructuring.

(4) The tendency of gender selection in AIDS susceptible population

As far as sexual transmission is concerned at least, the national random sampling demonstrates that, men exceed women with multiple sexual partners, which are likely to be HIV carriers. That is to say, women are mainly infected by others and passive victims. At the same time, since women are less likely to transmit the acquired HIV again, they objectively act as a "dam" to stop the spread of AIDS.

This situation fundamentally stems from the contradiction between the social reality of "male-centered cultural system" and the constitutional provision of equality between men and women. Therefore, the realization of gender equality is a positive social restructuring. Without this, it would be difficult to control the AIDS, what's worse, the "AIDS issue" might be one of the "gender war" fuses.

In addition, the phenomenon of "illness-resulting poverty" and "poverty-caused illness" will become prominent in the AIDS field sooner or later, thus becoming a better example of the "AIDS issue" originating from and acting on society.

(5) The timing of the high prevalence of AIDS

In recent years, some people, which see AIDS mainly from the perspective of disease, have repeatedly warned that China will soon see a huge epidemic of AIDS, and tend to exaggerate the imminence of high epidemic.

As the proverb goes, "to come early is not so good as to come in time". If the high prevalence of AIDS happens to coincide with some other serious social crises, then the two sides will form "mutual construction" and expand exponentially. In other words, we are not fighting against the "natural spread" of AIDS, but against the pace of other crises during social restructuring that may come. It is this issue that is truly enough to be raised to the political height of life and death.

(6) The changing meanings of the life risk caused by AIDS

Against the background of governments stressing the importance of representing the fundamental interests of the broad masses and constructing a harmonious society, the modern Chinese people and public opinion has started from the height of safeguarding right to subsistence to view the phenomenon of "people's death". Additionally, the concealed people's "fault" is revealed; the supremacy of individual life value is valued. Thereafter, those who die of AIDS will no longer be just individuals, but a part of the people. Thus, it is possible to investigate and affix the government's responsibility. This means that social managers should keep pace with the time to coordinate this important aspect of social restructuring.

1.1.4 Prospects for Solving the Problem: Promoting the Process of Social Restructuring in China

The AIDS issues is not only a mirror of social restructuring, but also subjects to the rhythms of that process. The most prominent example of this is "community-based AIDS prevention and treatment".

At the international level, people finally realized the importance of sociocultural factors in the spread of AIDS, and finally began to promote AIDS prevention and treatment based on the community as a sociocultural cell after a long period of practice from a medical perspective to a public health perspective and then to a behavioral (individual) perspective,

In China, however, the population distribution under the urban "unit ownership" and the traditional village communities in rural areas are all disintegrating rapidly, so the extent to which "community" exists in China is itself open to question. Therefore, the applicability of almost all the specific contents of the foreign success models cannot be overestimated in today's Chinese society. Examples such as "community leaders" and "community spiritual resources" are even more uncommon in the daily life of Chinese people. A considerable amount of urban grassroots work is institutionalized rather than communalized.

The root cause lies in the directionality of the most important social driven forces: economic development, institutional reform, changes in interpersonal relations and spiritual life. When these factors converge to a positive joint force, "community", "middle class" and "rational society", such beautiful things will emerge. But the opposite is more often observed in Chinese reality. This means that in China, it is not so much a question of how to function as a community as it is a question of how to get scattered individuals to form a community. Therefore, we must carry on the party's fine traditions of building communities and promoting social restructuring just as we mobilized the people, in order to provide a solid base for the fight against AIDS. Based on the same token, similar macro examples need our further attention.

The prevention operations against AIDS, for example, pay particular attention to the "migrant population" and regard it as as one of the most important channels of transmission, and many interventions have been made to it. However, in real life, "migrant population" has been far away from the original group and has not formed a new social component. Their position in the operation of the whole society is often not only "marginal" but also "beyond the bound".

In this respect, it is easy to pay attention to the so-called "migrant workers" who are neither workers nor farmers, but to overlook the similar situation of the "white drifter" (white-collar workers of all kinds) who are probably about the same number as the migrant workers. On the one hand, their contribution to social development is often confined to the pure economic significance or as a tool, and this is one of the important reasons for the shortage of social restructuring power resources. On the other hand, there is a tension between the differential social network and the pyramidal structure of the society. This situation calls for the necessity and urgency of social restructuring.

If we do not understand this kind of social restructuring or just neglect it, and still use the power of administration to prosecute publicity and education in the old way under the planned economy system, then it is very likely that even the people who should be educated will be difficult to find. The benefits of the following work will be difficult to predict. If so, the outcome of second-time spread of AIDS through the "migrant population" shall be attributed to the lack of timely social restructuring, the absent basic foundation for the prevention and control work, rather than simply the failure of the prevention and control work.

If we can move away from the traditionally pyramidal approach, and give more play to the role of social networks (an important aspect of social restructuring), then the impact of AIDS prevention and treatment efforts may be better than our expectation. Generally speaking, since AIDS is spread through social networks, this is the most effective way to prevent it.

For another example, AIDS prevention also attaches great importance to "peer education" among adolescents. But in real life in China, teenagers tend to contact "classmates" and "accomplices" (in a negative sense, "gang"), lacking the kind of "peers" with whom they can discuss sex, pregnancy, drug use and blood sales. As a result, a considerable amount of "peer education" in China tends to simply replace the lecturers from doctors with excellent classmates, while the content and emotional relationship of the lecturers remain basically unchanged, and its effect is greatly reduced.

Nor is it just a question of workers who conduct the prevention activities. Our society is beginning to realize that the twenty-first century Chinese youth need a new form of social cohesion outside the school system, such as online forums like BBS, Internet chat rooms, and "clubbing" (unexpected gathering).

In fact, teenagers have created or introduced these forms and started their own social restructuring. Adults should better help and guide them rather than suppress and regulate them, so as to reduce the incidence of "deviant behavior" in the "peer society" of teenagers. Otherwise, HIV prevention among adolescents is more likely to be in an "I need to do" manner rather than "I want to do". We should motivate these new combinations of young people to participate in social activities and even political activities, believing that their high patriotic enthusiasm will bring more vitality to China's development. Thus it makes the AIDS prevention and control more effective.

To sum up, life experience in history has taught us that SARS was mainly stopped by traditional administrative organizations (which is now taken as a successful experience), but that our "society" has not worked as expected. AIDS was then identified as a "matter of life and death", which provided a valuable historical opportunity for us to focus on social restructuring.

Since the beginning of the twenty-first century, the most significant change in Chinese society has been the unprecedented and consistent emphasis on the fundamental issue of "people" by all classes and walks of life. Therefore, it is no longer just a question of "preventing AIDS requires political participation". Instead, AIDS is moving towards a political issue at the level of social setting, for more and more people are beginning to realize that AIDS harms not only individual life and public health, but also the very fundamentals of a society. What is particularly pressing is that, expect for the debate over ideas, specific approaches to the fight against AIDS have caused and will cause greater social debate.

Many of the specific prevention efforts that have been permitted, supported and encouraged by the government are in fact in serious conflict with existing laws, social policies and moral precepts. Like, issuing clean needles to injecting drug users (conflicting with the regulations of compulsory drug addiction rehabilitation), promoting 100% condom use in entertainment places (violating laws and regulations of penalizing prostitution), encouraging gays to adopt prevention measurements (breaching the moral precepts), expanding and developing various non-governmental organizations (conflict with community law).

As a result, the question of whether necessary specific work of the prevention and treatment of AIDS will destroy our existing laws, morality, marriage, family system and spiritual civilization construction was raised among the general public and even among AIDS prevention and treatment workers.

In fact, the above phenomenon are regarded as "conflicts" and these conflicts can often be easily solved at the grass-roots level. It also involves the construction of some social forces and dedicated institutions, among which the most important is the "policy development" by the local top leaders. However, this is still not on the road of rule of law construction, nor enough to achieve sustainable development.

The leaders and guides of Chinese society have made a choice between forcing AIDS prevention work to conform to the current social setting and using the power of AIDS prevention to carry out social reform and even system reform. If the concern about substandard AIDS prevention and treatment has been mixed with efforts to maintain social stability and social system, then the urge that AIDS prevention and treatment must achieve its goals has permeated the will to promote social reform. This is the adequate understanding of "the highest political positioning".

In order to firmly implement it, we should do something from the perspective of social restructuring. For example, we can strengthen the supervision of those rent-seeking departments, and make it more difficult for them to seek rent, thus changing the "high-risk groups" of AIDS into "high-risk groups of victims" on the whole. We will empower them and support them to fight against the rent-seeking departments, and mobilize other social forces to actively participate, and so on.

From the point of view of building a harmonious society, we must ask the question as follows: compared with the harm of AIDS itself, the social loss caused by any possible error in the concept and operation of AIDS prevention and treatment is greater. We must avoid them in order to protect not only individual life, public health and social stability, but also the development of China's social restructuring and our future.

Generally speaking, our society should adopt the proposal of "construction force with human rights-orientation". Then, both the construction of AIDS issue and the practice of AIDS prevention and treatment will drive social restructuring in China.

To build new forms of social grouping on the basis of comprehensive interests of individuals. For example, a group of men at high risk of AIDS have spontaneously formed a reticular aggregation, which is different from the pyramidal organization; to encourage different "aggregations" to form social "merges" (rather than unified combinations) by contract (rather than by absolute struggle), as is already being done tentatively among the various AIDS nongovernmental organizations; to foster a well-acknowledged consensus (not vertical instillation) on the basis of pluralistic equality (rather than single indoctrination). For example, in the prevention of sexual transmission of AIDS, many successful programs rely on consensus among all participants (not executive orders) to move closer to the goal of "100% condom use". To encourage social management departments at all levels to re-examine and re-write all kinds of institutionalized content with the basic starting point of protecting human rights. For example, a series of such local laws and policies in some provinces have been successfully introduced and implemented.

Overall, in the current construction of AIDS and in the practice of AIDS prevention and treatment, some content of China's social restructuring and its development level have been reflected in the process, thus becoming a symbol of the development level. Moreover, because the "AIDS issue" has been constructed and established by the highest power at the highest political level, the use of this symbol in social research is probably the most visible and profound one.

It is from such a perspective that the so-called "AIDS issues" should be constructed from a positive perspective as "the best opportunity for social restructuring". By doing so, we can take AIDS as one of the breakthrough points and drive the re-construction and re-development of the whole society. Similarly, its construction of the human rights orientation and the correct guidance of AIDS prevention and treatment should be integrated into the process of China's social restructuring to achieve success.

1.2 Fear of AIDS: The Ultimate Weapon Against the Sexual Morality

Undoubtedly, education for AIDS prevention is indispensable and proper, but the key questions are as follows. First, what is the purpose of education? Is it actually for everybody's health or just for sexual morality? Second, which methods should be considered? Accurate scientific knowledge or hyperbolic panic?

1.2.1 Illnesses Are Always Reduced to Political Tools

In human history, any threats of illnesses could be greatly exaggerated for their own purposes by certain social forces under the kindest banner.

In the middle age of the nineteenth century, syphilis ran wild in western Europe. Under the guise of "medicine" and "disease prevention", some people launched a sustained campaign named "Social Purity Movement". In 1870s, Contagious Disease Acts was finally promulgated by the UK's government under the influence of these impellers. It was just crying up wine and selling vinegar. Everyone knew that it's actually a law on forbidding prostitution, behind which the real reason, rather for the sake of public health, is that the widespread prostitution and syphilis enormously eroded Navy and Marines' effective force for a few occasions of the British Empire's colonial expansion. In 1857, for example, when there was a large-scale rebellion in India, Britain failed to send reinforcements from its native land because of the syphilis.

However, history has witnessed the true hero who contained the syphilis. It was not such "Social Purity Movement" but the arsphenamine invented in the early twentieth century and penicillin in the 1930s. Ironically, the reduction of prostitutes was neither a result of this kind of repression, but its opposite—sex revolution, started in the 1960s. After the revolution, fewer men seemed to go whoring, so the business languished.

That was when AIDS was heard by Chinese. Sex revolution has started in China since the late 1980s. Anyone who had a little interest about the world knew its arrival in China. Few formal theories could criticize it back then and there was no seemingly viable measures to keep it at bay. Meanwhile, AIDS, once reported in the west, was immediately called by some Chinese with irony as "Acquired Illness from Dollars". Then several cases of HIV appeared in China. Though there were only a couple of cases, among which mostly were addicts, all the media desperately associated it with sexual morality (unfortunately until now, they still don't have sufficient evidence), as if they had hit the jackpot. The last hope for the purge of sexual morality all counted on this STD, which was why there was such a large-scale man-made "AIDS phobia". Yet, the influence was well beyond the actual incidence of AIDS. Some might even exclaim that only monks and nuns are safe!

Unfortunately, international studies have long shown that the more people feel panic, the quicker they are to recognize its falsehoods, and become more complacent or nonchalant than before. AIDS panic will soon end up like this. Even today, scaremongering does little to prevent AIDS but only makes its spread easier.

1.2.2 Panic is Bound to Aggravate the Spread

Imagine if a farmer in a southern border region were infected with HIV. What could he do under the present "AIDS panic"? All the neighbors would stay away from him. Not only would they refuse to shake hand with him, but to talk to him (actually neither of these spread AIDS). No one would ever go to the bathroom or touch any of the dishes he used (mere skin contact doesn't spread AIDS either). He would be restrained from working in township enterprises or taking part in any collective activities. Even tilling in his own fields might be watched, lest he might step on others' lands. Some might persuade his wife and children to leave him, and even quarantine his wife and children like they do to him. As a result, he had to leave home, using a false identity. Even if the government imposed a mandatory quarantine on him, it's not jail time. He could easily escape if he wanted to. In a new place, he would definitely bury his secret and might have sex again with someone else without condom. On top of that, he might sell blood without scruple and share the same syringe for drugs with someone else. And his wife might get pregnant and give birth. In this way, through body fluids transmission, he transmitted HIV to a new region.

While the virus would not happen to another region, if, on the other hand, his former neighbors had knew that AIDS was virtually in-transmissible without body fluids; If they weren't so panicky and jittery, harmoniously living together would not be a matter.

It's that simple. People who have been infected for any reason are just patients, not criminals. Panic can only lead them to conceal the truth, refuse inspection, isolation, and education, and then flee away. Some may even resort to retaliatory action against the society. If we really want to control and prevent AIDS, isn't scaremongering shooting ourselves in the foot?

For the sake of prevention, instead of sparing money to scare everyone, it's better to focus on those "high risk" groups; instead of vainly counting on that fear will deter teenager from having less sex, encouraging them to use condoms is more practical; instead of letting the government deal with the problem, ending up undermining its prestige, it is better to mobilize the civilian forces to achieve class restraint and community restraint; instead of taking carriers as "public enemies", let's simply treat them as patients.

I highly doubted the use of AIDS panic to purge sexual morality. AIDS is just a viral disease, whose cause and transmission routes are very clear. It will certainly be much easier and sooner to conquer AIDS than cancer. By then, will there be any other weapons to purge sexual immorality?

1.2.3 Argument Against Our Present Understandings of AIDS Patients

There is no doubt that many people infected with AIDS are resulting from immoral behaviors. If we do not face up to this point, we cannot convince others simply by taking the examples of farmers selling blood. But why should you understand those unethical behaviors?

What needs to get across is simple: either AIDS or flu is just a kind of disease; The infected are all patients; We should treat all of them equally. In other words, what's important is the patients' conditions, not reasons behind it. Otherwise, how can we be sure that among those who have the flu, no one is infected by kissing a mistress? Is it because the doctors understand "keeping a mistress" so they'd like to treat him? Or should a doctor first understand this behavior before treating him?

Illness is illness, which requires treatment. Judgment against patients' identities is not acceptable; Otherwise, prison doctors are totally needless, for it's better to let criminals die of illnesses. Likewise, the cause shouldn't be a determinant either, or doctors should perform like a vice squad—investigate into the patient first and then make the decision.

I'm sure no one hopes for this. Except saints, almost everyone has done something unethical at one time or another. But should it be the reason for the ignorance of our illnesses? However, getting sick is one of our most basic personal rights.

1.2.4 The Proper Understanding

The so-called "understanding" is actually an attitude between opposition and support. Who says that one should support or even learn about unethical behavior just because one understands it? "Understanding", shown by a small number of role models, can be close to infected patients; But for ordinary people, treating them equally is more than enough.

Were my acquaintance infected with AIDS, I should help him for medical treatment as same as I would do for flu patients, instead of dodging him like a plague or even expecting him to die. If AIDS were found in my neighborhood, I may not be able to help, but there is no need to kick them out. Nor would I unjustifiably ask the government to eliminate them. If I had a say in the decision, I would never have made a ridiculous rule like "no swimming pool for AIDS patients". AIDS is not contagious in that way.

In a word, it is not hard to understand them, once you know how AIDS spreads. By then, you will not frighten and quarantine yourself or treat the patients as criminals and could lend a hand when they need. Only in this way, in this so-called "AIDS era", can one enjoy a comfortable life. The number of AIDS will undoubtedly increase and then what should I do? Should I escape to the moon?

I have done a survey in a region where AIDS had been found. Most people there believe that the patients should be locked up in an isolated place. Why, some lamented, has not the government done anything yet?! Someone volunteered to pay and help, and some even had picked up a place for the "jail".

Perhaps, in reality, the idea of establishing the "AIDS Concentration Camp" prevails more than the incomprehension of the disease. As the cases increase and expand, the idea will not only become more universal but also more influential, which needs further discussion. For, it is not merely a matter of ignorance anymore, but a basic problem pertinent to the ways with which people get along.

The rationale of the "AIDS Concentration Camp" is that infected people endanger others, and that anyone who does harms should at least be locked up. If the government does not take any action, the harmed are supposed to do so. That is how all the "lynchings" and illegal detentions happened, often with plentiful supports. Does it make sense? Let's use our common sense.

First, how did I get a flu? It must be given to me by someone else. If I were to punish him, people would say that he didn't mean to it, which indicates that unintentional infecting behavior does not accordingly vest me with the right to punish the carrier. It's nothing but a necessary price to pay for living in this world. In this case, how could I be so sure that all HIV carriers definitely infect others on purpose?

Second, if I only call for patients who get sick first in a flu season to be grounded, but fail to take prevention, people will think I'm stupid. In particular, not everyone gets sick, even in the worst flu season. That is to say, the so-called cost is often very easy to avoid. Consequently, if I can take precautions but still demand the establishment of the "AIDS concentration camp", I'm bullying the weak.

Third, even if I were infected by someone deliberately and were able to kill him/her, would I be cured therewith? Obviously, I'm just venting my anger. And how could that be justified as the AIDS patients' spite deserve to be punished. Does their illness come out of nowhere? Therefore, if that happens, the dispute will be endless. The shared security will be ruined.

Fourth, as a citizen, I certainly have the right to ask the government to protect me, and so do the AIDS patients. Especially, when my right is at the cost of others', will I still be so assured? In this era, after the entrance of WTO, if I have yet to understand what "all men are equal", negotiation and win–win situation mean or what "live with others peacefully" is, I suppose I am not entitled to tell the government how to do.

In general, for example, why there is a difference between the attitudes towards the snake—in the past, letting a snake escape without killing it is considered immoral, but now the snake becomes a dish and even has legislative protection as a pet. For our humans have no longer blindly fearing and wiping out things that we can easily prevent and come to understand that every bell we toll for others is ringing for us as well; Man is coming across that there can be no more enemies on this one and only earth. The only way to obliterate all enemies for ever is to make them friends.

In the end of April 2001, I called on a moribund AIDS patient infected by selling blood in a county. He was a poor peasant whose home had nothing but bare walls, lying in the only decent wooden bed waiting for death. His five other family members—his brother, two sons, daughter-in-law and son-in-law also infected by the blood sale—stood by him helplessly.

His son said, "My house is built by my father with his blood."

His brother said: "None of the relatives or friends came to see him. It makes no difference whether he lives or dies. We've already in another world." What worried the family most was that no one would carry his coffin.

I could not help taking hold of his bony hands. So I wrote these lyrics, hoping someone would compose for it. Let's sing to show our care for the infected. At that time, I went with three certificated doctors in charge of the work of AIDS prevention and control. None of them entered the house, except an administrative official. But he did not shake hands with the infected. After I left the house, the three doctors gossiped, "After all, he is not professional". That's why I was urged to write the song below.

Couldn't Help Holding Your Hands—Cares for All AIDS Fighters

Couldn't help holding your hands

My strange friend

Your innocence fills me with guilt in mind

Long apart, you and I

I've been lost in mediocre life

Original aspiration was left behind

While upon the duty is shouldered on mine

Couldn't help holding your hands

My close friend

Your suffering is the wound of all men

Forgive me my friend, longing to hold you tight though I can't

But the story remains for which each name stands

Please don't say you are running out of time

Humanity like bright blooms always shines

Couldn't help holding your hands

My unforgettable friend

Shedding tears will not be my only act

Life has changed and will never turn back

Empathy, unity

And fraternity will save us out of the jam

Life has changed and will never turn back

Excuses to retreat should be abstained

Caring first the fate of people and then of mine

And love will never berth on the bank

1.2.5 The Social Significance of the Fight Against AIDS: A Responsibility for the Lives of Citizens

The acute spiral of AIDS spread in China alarms that we are running out of time.

It would be overstated to say that the Chinese government has not fully realize the enormity of this threat. But when it comes to specific problems, government's efforts are often resisted, or even dismissed, by muddle-headed views, especially concerning the attitudes towards sex workers.

It's acknowledged that if one uses condoms every time in contact with sex workers, it is difficult for AIDS to spread to other populations. Therefore, one of the major efforts to prevent AIDS worldwide is to promote 100% condom use among sex workers. Chinese government has, in fact, fully endorsed this approach and has begun to pilot it.

Many, however, yelled, "It's condoning and supporting prostitution!" As a result, the government seems a bit like doing an underground work.

First, it is, above all, an ostrich policy. Even if we assure that we can completely eradicate the illegal "sex industry" in China within five years, will AIDS spare us five years? Do people dying of AIDS by sexual transmission during this period deserve it? And who can assert when the "sex industry" will be rooted out? It will be a historical responsibility.

Second, the argument is illogical. Promoting 100% condom use is not contradictory to the "anti-pornography". Still less does it mean that the "sex industry" will be legalized accordingly. They totally can go hand in hand. For instance, to manage cities' appearance, on the one hand, there will be rules against littering, and on the other hand, the government will spend money in hiring a large number of cleaners. Does the employment of cleaners indicate tolerance and support for littering? Or as long as the rules against littering exist, cleaners will be unnecessary?

Third, the idea is utterly impractical. It assumes that if prostitution were safer, more people would do it, or that the current AIDS threat could cripple the sex industry.

In fact, it's totally groundless. The global rate of condom use has surged since the "Age of AIDS", but there has been no significant decrease or increase in any form of unethical sexual relationships. The reason is simple: no sexual relationship, including prostitution, is determined only by a single factor: sickness. Besides, has there ever been a single cause for anything in this world?

My overall impression on the "sex industry" after years of is: STD and AIDS would have frighten those to death who at first are impossible to go whoring. While those who have been involved in are basically not afraid, because the dozens of extremely realistic hidden motives and reasons are more important than "getting sick", and more urgent. The single most acceptable thing for them to do is to use condoms, rather than to "abstain from immorality" for fear of getting sick.

Fourth, the statement is just a glimpsed view of the entire forest. If AIDS is merely transmitted between the client and the hooker, the problem will be much easier. But what did the client's wife or girlfriend and the street girl's husband or boyfriend do wrong? Why should we stand by and watch them harmed by AIDS? Moreover, AIDS will be transmitted sexually from them to thousands of ordinary people who have no connection with the "sex industry". And how do they do wrong?

Fifth, it's simply irrational. In daily life, everyone knows the truth of "choosing the lesser of two evils". Why people become irrational when it comes to the "hooker"? It's true that the "sex industry" threatens social decency, but AIDS is deadly!

Sixth, such a statement puts the responsibility of government last. Why does the government want to crack down on pornography? It is not because of the animosity towards hookers, but because the government believes that the campaign against pornography can maintain social decency and objectively protect the people's interests. But what interests could be more precious and more important than human life? Therefore, the government is now promoting 100% condom use, putting human life first. What's wrong with it?

Finally, I have to point out that the reason why this view is so inveterate and popular is actually derived from a deeper idea: it is better for immoral people to die! Some even call it “racial cleansing”.

I don’t bother to refute this kind of idea, and only two points will suffice. Firstly, in this case, you censure others immoral; but on another issues someone else may denounce you immoral. In consequence, should it be better for you to die as well? Secondly, your opinion is your own affair; Why on earth should the government do the same? The hookers and clients are also human beings. While the government performs their management duty, they also spare no efforts to protect health and lives of the public, which exactly embodies the government’s comprehensive responsibility for the public. Will you object to a government like this?

1.3 The Values of AIDS Prevention and Control in China

AIDS prevention and control in China has been carrying on for 30 years, in which the research of humanities and social sciences has long been joined and has yielded fruitful results. However, the researches is mainly focused on specific issues, and the rare panoramic researches are often limited to the cause itself, lacking into its social and historical sources and the social role it plays.

In this chapter the cause will be put, as a whole, within the framework of Chinese societies’ overall development process. It’s supposed to reveal that as the soul of many specific works, what kind of changes has the values been through, what is the functional mechanism behind it, in the contemporary history of China what role does it play and what luminous and far-sighted significance it brings.

1.3.1 Political Values: From “Defense” to “Taking Responsibility” and then to “Rights Protection”

When AIDS was first discovered in China, a social trend caught on which believes that AIDS is actually an “Acquired Illness from Dollars”, one of the manifestations and products given rise by the invasion of western ways of life. It advocates “keeping the enemy at bay”. But this unconscious hangover of the old class struggle was transient and quickly reversed in the late 1990s. The most important impetus has come not from the spread of scientific knowledge, nor from the voluntary correction of governments and societies, but from three seemingly unrelated social changes.

The first change took place when China’s economy started to take off. Especially after the entrance of WTO, the cognition of globalization of Chinese government has quietly shifted from the simple view of merely “opening up” gradually to the second stage—the “global village”, a concept based on interdependence and mutual development. Therefore, it could be understood that the turning point in the cause of

AIDS prevention and control in China at the end of the twentieth century, when the "defense theory" was completely abandoned, was driven neither by the international community nor the specialized department World Health Organization, but by the World Bank, an official organization of sovereign states. Especially since then, the Chinese government has fully opened its door to the comprehensive work of international agencies (including non-governmental organizations) for AIDS prevention and control in China.

Meanwhile, a second shift has occurred. The daily life of Chinese people has taken a qualitative leap, which is not only in the substantial improvement of the material standard, but also in the emergence of the main characteristics in a consumption era in a broad sense. This leap impels the social mentality more prone to secularization, and to a large extent eliminates most of the previous political discourse, especially the kind of expressions used by struggle class during the Cultural Revolution. In consequence, the theory of "defense" failed to achieve its goals, and instead invoked widespread disgust and disdain, which subsequently lost its ground and laid a foundation for the correct understanding of AIDS prevention and control in the future.

The third change is that in the last decade of the twentieth century, sexual culture in China has undergone a revolutionary upheaval. Although the objective quantity of various non-traditional sexual relations and sexual behaviors may not necessarily soar, they are increasingly well known and even taken for granted in the public opinion. In the context of the low AIDS epidemic at that time, in the social psychological atmosphere where the change of "sex" was becoming more and more commonplace among ordinary people, the theory of "defense" was reduced to the ineffective intimidation of "the Wolf is coming", thus destroying its own foundation.

Since then, in the twenty-first century, the Chinese government has successively issued a series of major policies on AIDS, showing great political initiative, among which the most important one is the "Four Exemptions and one Care" policy for HIV-infected persons and patients in 2004 and the Regulations on AIDS Prevention and Control issued by the State Council in 2006. At the same time, the top leader of the state and the Party have been visiting the infected and patients on World AIDS Day for many years, exerting irreplaceable political influence. In particular, the Party School of the CPC Central Committee and Party schools at all levels have consecutively carried out training for AIDS policy, which not only elevated the cause of AIDS prevention and control to a political task, but also turned its executor into the party's top leadership. It should be said that such level of political attention is incomparable, even as to the attention to bilharziasis in the 1950s, let alone any other diseases. Even in other areas, it's rare.

It can be confirmed in review of these major measures that the Chinese government has raised the "AIDS issue" to the highest political level as "a concrete manifestation of China's great responsibility for the survival and development of the international community and human beings". It was mainly driven by three aspects. First of all, because the UN listed AIDS as the sixth of the Millennium Development Goals and the Chinese government, after the twenty-first century, hopes to become more involved in international affairs as a responsible major country. The second is the strong political demand for building a harmonious society at home. Third, higher political requirements for the top leaders were put forward during the development of the cause itself.

It means that the Chinese government is more consciously assuming political responsibility and a series of derivative responsibilities on the issue of AIDS prevention and control. This willingness to take responsibility in the field of AIDS is all the more extraordinary when compared with the government's constant emphasis on decentralization in the economic sphere and the same tendency in the reform of the health system. Notably, while the Chinese government is in charge, there is no obvious tendency of power centralization, but an increasing trend of decentralization. This kind of responsible but not centralized mode provides China's realpolitik a possible direction for development which deserves much attention.

Since the twenty-first century, many researchers and practical workers in the field of AIDS prevention and control have constantly raised the issue of "rights", including not only the individual rights of infected persons and patients, but also the rights related to or associated with all relevant groups. This kind of cognition and voice accumulate over time, and finally formed a strong public opinion in recent years. Although there is no definite affirmation in the official discourse, in the actual work of government agencies and institutions at all levels and of all kinds, safeguarding the due rights and interests of relevant personnel or groups has become a common practice, and has increasingly become one of the important subjects of AIDS prevention and control. So far, the Chinese government has not formally demurred this trend. The importance of this situation lies in the objectiveness of this development possibility: first of all, in this only field of AIDS prevention and control, the government takes a step further towards greater political responsibility of rights protection, at least not to deny the responsibility; and then they apply it to the whole process of social development.

1.3.2 Social Concepts: From "Departmental Cooperation" to "Social Mobilization" and then to "Community as the Main Body"

AIDS has been constructed as a social issue from the very beginning. Although the basic consensus that "social problems should be solved by the whole society" has been circulated for many years, the responsibility for the specific implementation has undergone different phases.

Since the early 1990s, the idea of "multi-sectoral cooperation" in response to AIDS has been the dominant idea of the government. It was regarded as a panacea at that time, but in fact, only a hangover of the "all-round government" in the previous planned economy period, which violated the trends of division and professionalization in social management that had formed before. Instead, it led to an awkward situation as "no cooperation, no action" among the departments. In particular, this kind of opinion mainly emphasized the state power, which objectively impeded the participation of other social forces.

Up to the twenty-first century, a variety of social organizations have sprung up. They have achieved increasingly remarkable results in the practical work of AIDS prevention and control, especially the MSM organization. Furthermore, folk networks of organizations were formed and began to function as a social force. This progress coincided with the change of Chinese government in "purchasing social services", which promoted the national AIDS prevention concept to "social mobilization" and the government began to directly allocate funds to support all kinds of mass organizations concerned.

The shift is not trivial. It has gone beyond the struggle between "devolution and power centralization" in the early stage of reform and opening up, and shifted from the single idea of "strengthening leadership" to the intention of implementing systematic project. The governing philosophy behind it can be concluded into four basic points: Recognize the existence of a relatively independent society and its various representative forces outside the government; play its role under controlled conditions; make certain acceptable concessions if necessary; challenge to the government's authority is absolutely not allowed. Although the implementation of this new concept, "social governance" can't be ascertained that it first appeared in AIDS prevention and control, it has been most fully demonstrated in this field, and can even be called unique. The progress of AIDS policy in recent years is largely due to the active participation of social organizations.

If the idea of social mobilization means the emphasis of the government on the reliance of the community as a base, then it gears up the widespread of the concept—"make community a main body", prompted by some social organizations. There are also four points in its main content, which almost correspond to the government's new idea of social governance.

First, it points out that relatively independent communities should be the main actors in the fight against AIDS, while the executive branches of the government should be a supporter or only a service provider. Second, the role played by the community is the most important and decisive driving force. Third, the work of government is not just to absorb communities, but to fully empower them. Fourth, the community subject and the government authority can totally help each other and achieve a win-win situation.

So far, the Chinese government, at least in the field of AIDS prevention and control, has not directly denied the new thinking mode of "make community as the main body". Its think tank has not only affirmed the remarkable results it has brought, but also proposed it as a policy of sustainable development. Theoretically speaking, there may be some tension between social governance and community subject. In practice, community struggles did happen, but as the "win-win" thinking mode becomes increasingly popular today, obviously, the two parties are more likely to develop under the continuous coordination and co-adaptation in the practice. The new resultant force formed in this process is bound to push the cause to a better new stage, and creates the possibility of leading the development direction in other aspects of the society.

1.3.3 Cultural Concepts: From "High-Risk Groups" to "De-stigamatization" and then to "Individual Rights Assertion"

In the early stage of AIDS prevention and control, the publicity and education of AIDS was centered around the concept of "high-risk groups" and even entangled itself, and there was a tendency towards insecurity among everyone. This way of thinking deliberately expanded the standards and methods of behavior in the specific work of public health into the classification and characterization of individuals and groups in the sense of social stratification, which objectively provides a theoretical basis for the epidemic of AIDS discrimination. This is no longer a mere theory of "defense", but a deteriorated theory of "seeking for enemies" or even "making enemies", which was one of the main reasons for the ineffectiveness of the cause in the early stage.

With the development of the two aspects mentioned in this section, practical workers, researchers and the public have increasingly discovered the serious harm of this fallacy, and started to fight back, directly promoting the social trend and practical action of "de-stigmatization" at the beginning of the twenty-first century.

In addition to the great achievements in the field of AIDS prevention and control, the social trend of "de-stigmatization" has served as impetus to the overall development of China. It has been popularizing deep-going new ideas of four levels to the Chinese people. First, stigma is neither ancient nor natural, but is actively constructed by some social forces in order to achieve a certain value goal. Second, the stigma is not only a real behavior aiming at some people, but a way to directly suppress the whole personality and social status of some hated individuals or groups. Third, if stigma is allowed to wreak havoc, certain social forces will be indulged to seize unlimited power, which will ultimately harm anyone and everyone. Fourth, "de-stigmatization" represents a great improvement of the overall civilization of a nation and a process of building the basic norms of interpersonal relations in modern society.

In the specific process of "de-stagmatization", each changes mentioned in this chapter has played its indelible role, but the most fundamental driving force is the trend in diversification of the emerging values and individual choices in the daily life of Chinese people since the twenty-first century. The unprecedented opportunity and feasibility of personal freedom for the Chinese in the private domain are forming a diffuse and colorful pattern of social life that is eroding the foundation of any stigmatization day by day.

In spite of all kinds of maladjustment and even panic, in social reality, the mainstream does not obviously oppose this kind of diversification of real life. Neither the Chinese government nor the dominant ideological force has made a clear statement upon it. This gives the idea of individual rights, at least in daily life, a corresponding living space and opportunity for development. It focuses on social campaigns for equal rights of all "sexual minorities", leading the way in the fight against AIDS. It was either a relief or a sudden rise; It may be targeted or flourish or it may run on its own course.

1.3.4 Life Notions: From "Keep Your Integrity" to "Participate in the Society" and then to "Take Civic Responsibility"

It has been closely related to the daily life of almost all Chinese people since the cause of AIDS prevention and control was launched in China. In the early days, Chinese people were freaked out by the publicity of 100% fatal rate and that the patients would die as soon as they were infected. As a result, the early AIDS prevention propaganda, no matter how scientific and accurate, was eventually distorted by some social forces into a single advocate of "keep your integrity".

The plausibility of the idea fooled a generation of Chinese, including scientists, and to this day has been criticized only for its impossibility. In fact, the idea has three fatal flaws. First of all, it advocates the subtext of "a quiet conscience sleeps in thunder", which suggests that the infected and risk actors deserve the punitive result, giving a green light to social discrimination. Secondly, it implicates a negative self-preservation attitude that mind your own business and others are none of your business, which is not conducive to mutual assistance among the people. Last but not least, it denies that people can be infected even if they preserve their integrity, making it easier for "honest people" to ignore the risk of AIDS.

Although there have always been people who believe firmly in the concept of preserving one's integrity, in the twenty-first century, driven by the changes mentioned in this chapter, more and more individuals, communities, social organizations and social groups begin to participate more actively in the prevention and control of AIDS. "Participation" becomes the strongest voice. In particular, this involvement has expanded from what began as simple advocacy to various forms of care and support aimed at various groups, such as AIDS orphans, infected persons, addicts, sex workers, homosexuals, etc. In many aspects, it's bigger, more pervasive and more relevant than any other social assistance.

In the process, the infected and the so-called "high-risk groups" themselves have become rising stars. The most distinct difference between them and other social organizations is not only that they are closer to the main body of the community, but also that they consciously regard "policy advocacy" as one of their important tasks. This originally refers to all kinds of suggestions from specific operators of public health to superior leaders. While domestic social organizations, especially civil organizations, have successively regarded themselves as the subject of behavior clearly and expanded the target to the national leadership and the whole society under the help of international forces. Although they are still toddlers and have to go through the process of grinding an iron pestle into a needle, these people and their groups, who until recently were only regarded as "sources of infection", can now participate as subjects in the decision-making process of leaders at all levels, or at least have the opportunity to express themselves to senior leadership. This is not only their growth and pride, but also a symbol of the transformation of the whole society. In particular, rather than rejecting them outright, the forces within the system have adopted quite a few of their policy recommendations, which are quite rare in other social areas.

In recent years, with continuous participation, people concerned have gradually begun to form a further consensus that participation is not only a social activity, but also a courageous and skillful undertaking to shoulder their civic responsibilities. The main points of this new consensus are threefold. First, every citizen, even the infected, has inescapable responsibility to the whole society, in addition to securing his or her rights. Second, this kind of civic responsibility does not constitute the power to control anyone else, nor does it constitute the neglect of the government's leadership, but more importantly, it is the sublimation of one's own public morality and civic personality; Third, civic responsibility is more about promoting social development than fulfilling it.

It is under the promotion of this consensus that in recent years, the intensity, breadth and depth of various social forces' planned participation in the cause of AIDS prevention and control has increased exponentially. Together with the leading role of the government, it has formed a two-way construction of "AIDS issues".

Such civic action and social participation not only bring good news to AIDS prevention and control, but also shouldn't be underestimated for China's overall social development. It indicates that the real "society" of China is gradually restoring, and the real "development" in China is more promising.

1.3.5 Core Concepts: From "National Salvation" to "Health" and then to "Happiness"

All the four changes above point to the same focus, namely that they have a core idea and have also undergone historical improvement. At the beginning of the emergence of AIDS, China basically followed the idea of "national salvation". The country's official attitude is "AIDS prevention and control concerns closely with economic development, social stability and national security and its rise and fall. It also concerns with national quality and state's rise and fall". And in the mass media, sensational call inundates everywhere. Almost everyone relevant are dashing towards exaggerating the hazards.

This kind of situation, at the very beginning influenced by lacking cognition, was still largely decided by the kind of tradition permeated in the blood of Chinese intellectuals (including technology experts) since the May 4th movement—"saving the nation from subjugation" as their own duty, as sacred ideal and as highest moral ground. It is not inherently wrong, but it is very easy to objectively ignore or even suppress intellectuals' unique value to society: rational thinking.

It was also linked with a special historical period in the last decade of the twentieth century when the intellectual class interacted with the political system. The professionals represented by science and technology experts not only controlled the discourse power of social fundamentals including the economy, but also had a tendency to "cross the boundary" and began to express their feelings straightforward and even inordinately. Meanwhile, the leadership was in the process of understanding the complexity of the society, so the two sides hit it off and jointly produced a kind of AIDS panic of national destruction.

Fortunately, history is honest. Although Chinese AIDS response is far from what it should be, and the spread is indeed expanding, the doomsday scenario has not yet come true. Driven by the changes described in this chapter, by the twenty-first century, the idea of "national salvation" began to recede, and not a cloud had been left behind.

The fundamental problem faced by the cause thereafter is no longer just how to do it, but why to do it; It's no longer just about resources, but about soul regeneration. In consequence, what idea should be taken as the core of cohesion and the guideline? At the mean time, humanities and social scientists are gradually getting involved in the Sino-British project. Professor Li Dun, the pioneer, began to preach the proposition to the senior leadership that "AIDS prevention and control is to realize individual right to health", raising the issue to the height of individual rights. Since then, despite the voices that it's much beyond the purview of public health and indeed a long march from advocacy to implementation, thus unworkable, the concept of health and the right to health spread faster and gain more and more recognition.

It all thanks to the keen and profound perception from humanities and social scientists of the pulse of the Chinese society. Since the twenty-first century, in a society where personal hygiene conditions, medical technology and living standards have been constantly improving, the old anxiety of "never get infected with any disease" has been decreasing. Meanwhile the new awareness of "it is difficult to buy health with money" has been ascending. In daily life of the civilians, "prevention" began to give way to "health care", "preventing from being sick" was replaced by "staying healthy", and even "seeing a doctor" was interpreted as not better than "doing exercise". Based on such social changes, humanities and social scientists abstracted the well-timed key word "health", which pointed to the focus of the times and the hearts of everyone, with the greatest appeal and cohesion.

The Chinese government quickly adopted the idea of health, not only using it as the core concept of AIDS prevention and control, but also consciously extending it to the broadest social sphere. The latest evidence is the enactment of the administrative regulations on the development of health services.

But the progress is never fast enough. A new page of the cause of AIDS was soon unfolded. In recent years, under the shock of the diversity of secular life, more and more people are looking for their spiritual home. But since the grand narratives in the past have been largely disintegrated, one has to find some measure of life's purpose that is appropriate and applicable in this world. Then the word "happiness" rapidly becomes a concept, a discourse, and a new core idea.

No matter how scholars discuss the connotation and extension of "happiness", everyone knows in daily life that the essential difference between "happiness" and any previous value slogan is that it is a completely independent "subject construction", a crystallization of personal inner feelings and the goal of spiritual pursuit, which can exist only in comparison. In particular, it is the pursuit of happiness that most widely inspires the greatest initiative in the commonplace life. The country's leaders are in the midst of a rapid process of adopting, digesting and refining the core concept of happiness, which is likely to serve as the main bond between the "Chinese dream" and personal life. It would further the cause of AIDS, bringing new recognition and a new cultural awareness that all risky behavior is not just likely to make you ill, but could completely destroy your happiness. All public welfare activities are not only promotions of education, but also a "blessing". The appeal of all infected people and related groups is not taking a candy from a baby, but a natural impulse to pursue happiness. All the country's preferential policies are not privileges to the infected, but conscientious help for all people to achieve happiness.

It's undoubted that none of the developments analyzed in this chapter are likely to be synchronized, much less linear. They were interspersed with a variety of social forces and even conflicts, and the ideological trends were also diversified and competitive. Nevertheless, as far as the mainstream of development is concerned, the core concept of AIDS prevention and control in China is indeed in the process of continuous innovation. The new concept of "happiness" is just like the rising sun. It has a great future and is likely to play a leading role in the development of the whole Chinese society.

If so, the possibilities of new methods to be brought up during the development of the whole society will be greatly increased.

Chapter 2
The Cause of AIDS Prevention and Control—A Romance of the Three Kingdoms

The so-called "*Romance of The Three Kingdoms*" indicates that the cause of AIDS prevention and control is not only the battle between medicine and disease, but also the interaction and mutual construction among the three forces in the society—volunteer groups (community groups) that serve people with AIDS, Centers for Disease Control (CDC) and hospitals that treat AIDS.

"No discord, no concord" best describes them. They were tangled up due to the spread of AIDS and became indispensable and complementary to each other around the main body of AIDS. Nonetheless, the three parties are in different social positions. On the one hand, different conflicts of interests are inevitable; On the other hand, they constantly push each other and even transform each other in the interaction, finally forming the current benign recycle.

From the perspective of constructivism, it is far from enough to just describe the current good situation. Only by exploring the specific process of its formation and development and reaching the state of "knowing it and knowing what it is" can we make more contributions to promoting the development of the whole cause. To this end, in this chapter I will elaborate upon this issue.

2.1 Bi-Directional Conflict of Action Logic: Tripartite Construction of AIDS Patients' Orientation Towards the Response

As a new branch discipline, AIDS sociology not only needs a macro perspective of state and society, but, in particular, needs a micro perspective of the infected and carry out in-depth study of these AIDS victims. As I said in the first chapter, the results of the current research of AIDS sociology in this aspect are not enough, to a certain extent, resulting in an "aphasia" of the infected.

However, infected persons are not isolated. Instead, they form the closest and most relevant interactions, or even co-structures, with volunteer groups (community

S. Pan, *The Social Construction of AIDS Issues*, A Sociological View of AIDS,
https://doi.org/10.1007/978-981-16-7519-5_2

groups), health workers and the Centers for Disease Control within the AIDS prevention and control system. In other words, the relationship between the three parties is very much like the "Romance of The Three Kingdoms", in which each two parties are tied up, share interests, change each other and consolidate into one.

This chapter will therefore focus on this aspect, which could be rarely seen in domestic literature.

2.1.1 *Why Do Infected People React Negatively?*

(1) Presentation of the problems

Great progress has been made in the fight against AIDS in China, especially with more infected people getting involved. However, for a long time, a high proportion of people with AIDS after diagnosis, avoid or resist the follow-up prevention and control work, causing great uncertainty for the epidemic control.

In the initial design of prevention and control work, such problems should not arise at all. State preferential policy, responsible doctors and compliant patients should logically make the course smooth. So why is negative coping orientation still present in infected people? Does it just derive from their unconsciousness ?

(2) Literature review

As for this, our national academic community carries out the research mainly from three aspects.

Firstly, it discusses how to eliminate social discrimination from the macroscopic perspective. But there is a logical contradiction in this train of thought. No policy for the whole society, no matter how carefully crafted, can fully adapt to the bizarre needs of all individuals. Therefore, for AIDS prevention and control work, anti-discrimination is actually not a technical problem because the aid is too slow to be helpful, but a dream of "all-round stability".

Secondly, many studies have discussed how to solve the specific difficulties faced by people living with AIDS. The researchers hoped to help them overcome all plights and participate in the prevention and control work. They also face an insoluble logical contradiction: people's spiritual needs are hard to be included. Otherwise, although the "Four Exemptions and One Care" policy has greatly promoted the participation of infected people, why does it still omit so many aspects?

Thirdly, the research focuses on humanistic care, quality of life, and various psychological support, intervention, counseling and nursing. However, it's also a discrepancy without any solution because such psychological intervention is carried out under the assumption that the infected people's psychological status has some kind of deviation. To them, however, such a situation is not only the logical conclusion of their own mental process, but also the result of their own subjective initiative. According to the survey, I found that the infected who have "escaped" from the prevention and control work, often escaped not only testing and treatment, but also this kind of "remolding activity".

(3) Research intention

The studies mentioned tend to regard the questions in this chapter simply and naturally as the result of discrimination, hardship, or psychological disorders. It seems to me that this kind of leapfrog one-way attribution is far from enough. Only from the perspective of relevant "tripartite" interaction and deepen and detail to the level of action logic of all parties can we obtain stronger explanatory power.

It is expected that this chapter will help the mainstream society to better understand how the coping orientation of infected people come into being in order to find better resolution.

(4) Concepts and perspectives of this chapter

"The three parties" here include the Center for Disease Control (policy implementer), relevant health care workers, and volunteer groups (community groups) serving people infected with HIV. All the three different subjects can exert impact on the coping strategies of the infected.

The "logic of action", corresponding to the "guiding idea", refers to the reasoning, explanation and orientation that are actually presented in practical activities. This concept is more concrete and profound than "behavioral logic".

In the "two-way conflict", one is that the guiding idea and the action logic contradict each other in either party; the other conflict is that the action logic of each side also contradict that of the other two. The two conflicts exist at the same time. The reason for using the concept of conflict is that according to the survey, I found that the situation contributing to the negative orientation of infected people is beyond the level of "contradiction" or "game".

"Coping orientation" refers to the orientation of the diagnosed patients' behavior in the face of a series of follow-up tests, medication, medical consultation, treatment and hospitalization, especially the decision tendency of whether to participate in the process or to "flee" or resist. This concept is more intentional and uncertain than "coping strategies".

"Co-construction" means that the coping orientation of infected persons is not only their own intention, but more importantly a result constructed in the conflict of the three parties.

(5) The starting point of the argument

The biggest non-medical problem for infected people, of course, is discrimination. This is not fictitious or exaggerated, but directly reflected in the specific micro-situation: the role of the infected people, fair treatment, doctor-patient relationship and individual sense of belonging. Otherwise, "discrimination" is "non-subjective" and has nothing to do with them, let alone directly lead to any coping orientation. This chapter is therefore devoted to the analysis of these four aspects.

This chapter is based on my interview records of about 200,000 characters from 27 persons within the three parties in a certain city. Due to the limited space, the specific content will not be quoted.

2.1.2 *Self-Positioning of Infected Persons and the Conflict of Their Action Logic*

(1) Social identity

In China, any discrimination against AIDS infected people is strictly prohibited in any government document or mainstream media. The guiding principle is that infected people are equal citizens. However, while the policy of "four exemption and one care" has played a great positive role, strange and contradictory action logic has happened among some policy implementers. Many infectious diseases are fatal, but why can't other diseases enjoy such generous preferential treatment? Is it a kind of privilege?

No matter what kind of explanations have been made by scholars, in the face of an increasing trend of "comparison" among the patients with other diseases (such as hemophilia acquired by blood transfusion), those performers have to develop a logic to justify that the country's unprecedented preferential policies is only a method to block the continued spread of AIDS and reduce the death rate.[4] This logical contradiction positions the social identity of the infected person as only a carrier of AIDS, a source of infection, or even a person of guilt. It takes the state's preferential policies merely as a humanitarian behavior, and as the treatment of wounded enemy soldiers. Its outward manifestation is the common occurrence of all kinds of dodging and perfunctory excuses.

Healing the wounded and rescuing the dying should be the guiding principle of medical staff without exception. However, if an infected person comes to see a doctor, especially when an operation is needed, some people's action logic will be that this is an additional risk and burden, so they will put forward various professional prevarication and perfunctory excuses.

If infected people are just ordinary patients, their guiding principle should be "survival is the top priority". While in reality, their action logic is more dynamic. When they are first infected, they tend to regard themselves as "nasty people". After entering the treatment stage, they start to regard themselves as "patients". After gaining the awareness of rights protection, they begin to strive to become "ordinary people". Eventually, a few of the outstanding ones come to see themselves as "supermen", as they become more and more brave in the fight against AIDS, like "disabled heroes". As a result, except a small number of infected people who considered themselves sick, all the infected always have contradictory action logics with the "first two types".

This is actually the "identity and function crisis" of the infected in social mobilization. Once the conflict breaks out in some situations, each party will be deeply hurt because they do not know or admit their logical conflicts, which in turn strengthens their logical conflicts and the tripartite conflicts.

(2) Life identity

Country's guidelines treat infected people as the weak in life, so the "Four Exemptions and One Care" policy is justified. Nonetheless, the behavior of some policy performers indicates that in their logic of action, the infected person is just a patient of illness and has no other identity. Therefore, it is easy for them to ignore other life needs of infected people, such as marriage, mobility and support, which are not urgently needed for prevention and control, but helpful to the implementation of the policy yet relatively troublesome. The behavior of some medical personnel also deviates from the guiding concept of treating patients and saving lives. They believe that AIDS is nothing unusual and any opportunistic infection is still AIDS and must be dealt with specifically. That's why there are many prevarications and rejections.

In the meantime, infected persons also stray from the general guiding philosophy of "cure the disease first" What they value most is their various life identities, and they often make various "excessive" appeals based on this, ranging from daily trifles to "punishing the discriminator". In particular, this chapter focuses on those "runaway" patients, whose action logic is that what we run away from home for is not avoidance of HIV testing and treatment, but a voluntary give-up of most cherished life identity and protection of our families. They feel that this is their most painful sacrifice, and that society should compensate for it.

Unfortunately, policy enforcer and health care workers seldom want to understand the action logic of infected people out of their own logic contradiction. Instead, they simply attribute it to the infected people's "irresponsibility" or even "intentional harm to others" which will in turn, lead to more "flight" and even rebellion.

(3) Discrimination—another logical contradiction

Goffman defines "stigmatization" as a certain "humiliating" characteristic of an individual in interpersonal relationships, which gives it an "impaired identity" and is therefore seriously demeaned in status.

But the definition is far from being comprehensive. The so-called discrimination or stigmatization is also one of the logical contradictions. For normal patients, the guiding principle should have been "Disease is nothing more than disease. Just treat it". But for AIDS sufferers, the action logic of those with discrimination is reversed. What matters is not whether AIDS is shameful but is that those detractors take "the infected" as the AIDS sufferers' top most, only and in mass identity. They seize this one point and demean them while ignoring other facts. All other roles and identities of the infected persons are eliminated, and any positive value generated by their other identities is obliterated. As a result, the infected person is no longer an equal member of the human race.

In the national will and medical ethics, discriminatory guiding principles are definitely inhibited; no policy enforcers or health care workers will ever acknowledge or register such thoughts; However, infected persons, who are more sensitive due to illness, can often deeply experience a kind of "banal discrimination"[5] from their specific behaviors, which will generate negative coping orientations.

(4) The coping orientations of the infected

Research finds that the above conflicts among policy enforcers, health care workers and infected people are actually ubiquitous, yet most of which end up with the shrinking of the infected in the face of difficulties. And these cases are always little known. But this exactly activates the darkest parts of infected people's emotions. Their coping orientations are more likely to lead to self-abandonment, avoidance of prevention and treatment and even revenge on society.

But increasingly, the opposite is also happening. As mentioned earlier, infected people can grow up as well. Positive emotions will be aroused in those who early identify themselves as "normal people" or "supermen" in face of discrimination. Not only do they suffer fewer harms, but they also have more coping orientations towards fighting against them, thus in turn "forcing" the improvement of prevention and control work. Even infected people who only identify themselves as "being sick" tend to follow the logic of "A critically ill patient tries everything" and attempt to find health care workers who do not discriminate against them, thus reducing conflicts. Only those who consistently see themselves as "nasty people" are more likely to develop negative coping orientations.

That is to say, in addition to the self-improvement of policy enforcers and health care workers, the initiative to undo the bad effects is also in the hands of the infected people who maintain the unremitting self-growth.

(5) Inspiration: start with the "weak links"

The punishment for "intentional transmission" by the law is turning infected people into enemies; asking infected people to participate too much in prevention and control work is to encourage them to act like saint. Because what policy makers and health care workers want most is "treatment" rather than "prevention". Both of these approaches are logical departures from the guiding philosophy of "equal citizens".

Therefore, the role of medical personnel has become the "weak link" in the whole prevention and control work. Just like You an Hospital in Beijing, which has been highly praised by the state, we should break through the barriers of sectoral interests, put more resources into treatment units, and promote their gradual transformation into "homes for the infected" with a focus on social services.

2.1.3 Different Action Logic Between Policy Makers and Infected People

(1) Summary

The conflicts in this respect are firstly shown between policy makers and infected persons.

"Four Exemptions and One Care" policy and its local supplements, which have played a great positive role, are unprecedented special discounts. But this policy does not make it clear of what is exactly its guiding belief, so logic conflicts may arise when some policy makers are facing the appealing of infected people. They privately believe that the country's policy has been rather preferential. Therefore, if infected people still do not satisfy, they are "restless", "ungrateful", or even maybe "jackasses". That is unfair not only to the country but also to decision makers themselves. This unfairness is likely to generate resentment of policy makers towards infected people, and in turn, is likely to amplify or exacerbate negative behaviour of infected people. For infected people, the guiding belief should be "showing gratitude" of traditional Chinese culture. However, the action logic of a large number of infected people is quite the opposite: these benefits, in fact, are to prevent them from spreading HIV to others, so participating in testing and treatment actually equals making contribution to the country. Therefore, the country should "help them to do the whole thing well", otherwise it is unfair to them. Some people with iatrogenic infections think they are "grievously unfortunate," and may even become "permanent creditors," feeling that the country, society and others always owe them something.

This logical conflict manifests itself in many details, such as being tested involuntarily, being inquired about sexual partners, getting drugs with difficulty, being tested time and time again, being overprescribed, getting improper drug combination, being provided with second—and third-line drugs without free, and so on.

Despite the increasing communication between decision makers and infected people, both sides are reluctant to or afraid to talk about the most fundamental but most emotionally triggered issues—"whether it is fair or not" and "which side suffers more unfairness". Especially there is no way to prevent such a conceptual argument from turning into a personal grudge. As a result, the problem could not be solved for a long time. Instead, it becomes the logic starting point for some infected people to refuse to take medicine and treatment, and continue to conduct high-risk behaviors.

In contrast, many infected people who are brave and good at communicating and even contending with policy makers and health care workers are those people who have been treated unfairly and should have run away. Although these actions may be mistakenly thought as personal revenge, they are more efficient and yield a better effect. Especially these actions not only benefit the infected people themselves but all the infected persons. For example, government has introduced some operating instructions which aim at pursuing equality in recent years. These instructions are also the products of the infected people's game.

(2) Enlightenment: "equity brings harmony."

One of the biggest misconceptions of policy makers are that they assume that infected people will "naturally" understand and acknowledge that they are altruistic. However, the "public" mentioned by the former is only the "commonality" in the pattern of interests, while the basis of HIV patients' action logic is the "fairness" in the real life.

Therefore, as for the policy implements I met when I conducted the survey, the reasons why they were praised and welcomed by the infected lay in not only their diligence, but their practice of reasoning. Correspondingly, infected people say: if they are reasonable, we should be more reasonable. Thus, the two sides are equal—treating each other equally and being honest. This interaction not only resolved many conflicts, but also attracted many infected people from other places to seek a shelter.

2.1.4 The Conflict of Logic Action Between Doctors and Patients

(1) Overview

If HIV-infected people and staff of testing, medical treatment and nursing implement their own guiding beliefs, then there should be general doctor-patient relationships, without any particularity and much more conflict. However, once some ordinary friction occurs, it will spontaneously escalate into a conflict, even a serious one due to the big difference of action logic between two sides.

In the guiding belief of medical staff, all patients must be treated without discrimination and will not change because of their different social background. Of course, AIDS patients are of no exception. But infected people hold the opposite idea. They emphasize that they need special treatment precisely because of their special identity.

If this conflict only involves trivial matters like keeping their privacy, both sides can coordinate with each other perfectly. But if infected persons need surgery or hospitalization, the conflicts break out. Because at this moment, both sides are unconsciously betraying their guiding beliefs and are practicing the opposite action logic. Some health care workers stop treating them equally. In reverse, they emphasize the great risk of being infected. So they often charge more for taking extra precautions, or even refuse to perform surgery or make them hospitalized. The logic in these actions isn't right: the transmission routes of AIDS are actually far less than many other infectious diseases, so the general protection is sufficient. If the general protection is not in place, we can say that it is health care workers' negligence and we should not blame infected people who come to seek for medical attention.

However, this wrong logic seems to be quite prevalent. There are quite a few papers devoted to the self-protection of health care workers concerned, as if AIDS could be transmitted very easily. Some infected people have also deviated from their guiding beliefs. Instead of claiming that they are special, they begin to emphasize that they are just ordinary patients who do not need additional protection. Thus, they should not be charged with additional fees, let alone being rejected to have a surgery or hospitalization. This action logic contradicts with many special benefits that infected people actually enjoy. But this is the reason why many infected people take negative coping measures.

More importantly, neither side has learned enough lesson from it, and neither is willing to make its internal and mutual logic conflicts public. To a large extent, this misleads again.

Medical workers, not only those concerned but also likely to involve the whole group, often feel that "risking their own life to save others" is impossible and should not be done. Thus, they may question or even resist the preferential policies of our country, which in turn, is likely to lead to more professional excuses and denials.

At the same time, many infected people have a clear understanding of the grievance of the medical staff in their daily contact. They not only anticipate the "professional resistance" of some medical staff, but also are more deeply aware of their professional knowledge disadvantages in such conflicts. As a result, at least some of those infected have begun to travel far to other cities for treatment.

Just considering the above conflicts as it stands, both parties claim to be right. Therefore, I would like to remind the following enlightenment aiming at the integrated prevention and control work. A large number of scholars have suggested that AIDS should be gradually treated as a general chronic infectious disease as it is increasingly being controlled. But for policy enforcers, medical workers and infected people, it is no less than a reversal of fortunes, likely to trigger a new round of combat in the mode of Three Kingdoms.

For policy makers, if they regard AIDS as "chronic diseases" or even normal condition in the current environment which emphasizes the livelihood of people increasingly, no one can afford such political costs in the current environment which increasingly emphasizes people's livelihoods. For health care workers, this means there is no excuse to shrink. For infected people and community groups, abandoning the current special concession would be like cutting their own wrist. As a result, the three sides once again have two-way conflicts of action logic in the course of progressing and its disastrous effects are around the corner.

Of course, the situation is not all doom and gloom. Many of those infected have evaded testing or treatment. But the long and painful course of AIDS often forces them to think twice, only making them more adept at using various folk strategies. The action logic, which is to try to develop the doctor-patient relationship on the level of public affairs into one-to-one private communion, is always the same. For this reason, although I have heard constant complaints from infected people, I have been unanimously recommended by them to interview the medical staff who treat them like family members. Unfortunately, this approach to solve conflicts runs into with the social mobilization of "reorganizing medical ethics and forbidding private affairs", forming a "crevice blow". It is really regrettable.

Of course, there are many great men among policy makers and health care workers, for they are well known and will not be repeated here.

(2) Revelation: "Master and disciple are like father and son"

To resolve the above-mentioned conflicts, we will just get a drop in the bucket if we continue to rely only on policy enforcement or moral advocacy.

In the survey, one infected person said: "I have read all articles about AIDS on the Internet before I went to see a doctor. A doctor is no more than a teacher. How can they say I'm insatiable when I make a request?".

The words are simple but the sense is clear. Replacing doctor-patient relationship with master-disciple relationship will reduce conflict, truancy, and AIDS.

2.1.5 Individual Belonging: Different Action Logic Among Three Parties

The importance of belonging has been discussed by many scholars. However, in the study of HIV-infected people, the concept has not been independently proposed, but is scattered in areas such as social care or mental health. The term of "back to society" is usually used. My shows that this issue is significantly critical for infected people. Thus, it needs separate chapters and in-depth analysis.

(1) Where to belong

To this question, the guiding belief in the national policy is quite contextual. In the policy of "Four Exemptions and One Care", the country tends to see infected persons as an independent social group with strong commonalities, which should and can be treated separately. However, when advocating "multi-sectoral cooperation", the country tends to put infected people under a kind of "governance consortium". When speaking to the level of "social mobilization", the country pins its hope on social organizations, communities or social groups to accommodate the infected. When referring to medical care, the country tends to put infected people into patient group.

This can easily make many policy executors go their own way and develop a variety of deviant action logic. For example, some work units reject infected people. The reason is that they do not allow infected people to have jobs in their company, but they do not prohibit them to find another job in other place, so this does not violate infected people's corresponding rights. Many health care workers refuse with the same excuse: AIDS is infectious and we do not have the ability to accept and treat you. In other words, neither those decision makers nor those health care workers acknowledge that infected people should belong to them. But where infected people belong to is not a question perplexing them.

The action logic of infected persons about their belongings is more complex. Thus, we need further analysis about it.

(2) Rupture of intimate relationships

As the saying goes, "only full brothers can fight tigers, and only father and son can repulse enemies." That is to say, when we are in a more perilous situation, we need to depend more on domestic affections. However, infected people are encountered with a logical conflict and have to give up their most needed home because of the following four reasons.

First, with the exception of those iatrogenic infections, most of the infected cannot prove they are morally innocent. Second, they therefore do not have enough reason to seek for understanding of their partners, families and friends. Third, even if their relatives and friends discriminated against them seriously, they could not blame others. Fourth, they often abandon their homes and businesses and go away, but it is more difficult for them to find a new residence than the ordinary floating population, so they have to hide their illness.

As a result, some infected people form such action logic: they hate themselves, but they have nobody to tell and no way to alleviate. Then these emotions can explode anytime. In recent years, there have been many rumors about infected people "taking revenge on society". This suggests that this is one of the inevitable consequences of their lonely and depressed situation.

Although policy makers and health care workers have always been calling for improvement on aforementioned conditions, they feel powerless or inefficient because they cannot put their guiding beliefs into action.

(3) The puzzle of "regenerative home"

In recent years, many community groups have played a great role in taking care of and curing infected people, and also attracted and gathered a large number of infected people. The key word of their guiding belief is self-help.

The action logic of infected people participating in group activities is very clear—they want to find a sense of belonging, from obtaining various services, to gaining understanding and respect, and finally to "looking for home" and "being a decent person", etc. Such action logic is not only colorful, but also often multiple and dynamic.

As supporters and funders, the guiding beliefs of national or foreign funds are "social mobilization", aiming to comprehensively improve the living conditions of infected people. However, the action logic of many policy executors is usually limited to an utilitarian low level of "managing the infected", and thus, the guiding belief is diluted.

One of the most important and prominent guiding beliefs are mandatory testing. Since only community groups can gather masses of infected people, policy enforcers and foreign public welfare agencies often explicitly or implicitly require community groups to conduct as many tests as possible. They directly or indirectly make this as a condition of funding, or even to pay according to the people tested. If community groups accept this action logic, it must hit or even replace community groups' "home" activities to a large extent, making at least some of the infected feel that they are cheated again and taken advantage of again. Therefore, they will go away. The more serious the conflicts become, the more awesome the consequences are.

The infected often put the responsibility of such logical conflict directly on to the conveners of community groups. They thought that "we like him but hate what he does". This further creates logical conflict within the infected, which becomes the primary reason for weakening the cohesion of community groups.

In particular, although many community groups have good relationships with health workers, the active participation of the latter is often hampered due to various institutional barriers.

(4) The block of belonging

In addition to the main reasons mentioned above, there are four logical conflicts that discourage the enthusiasm of infected persons to participate.

First, what about sexual relations? The first guiding belief of sexual relationships is mutual trust. But most of infected people do not want others to know about their infection in order to avoid kinds of troubles that will follow. This is virtually impossible within community groups. Outside groups, infected people's infection is likely to be exposed for participating group activities. The result is that, contrary to the guiding belief of "informing your partner actively" in the mainstream society, "saying nothing" is the action logic prevalent among infected people.

Second, no matter how good a community group is, it will never substitute the role of family. On the contrary, it lets some infected people feel more lonely and helpless when they go back at night. So it is better not to participate and be stimulated.

Third, as regenerative home, the guiding belief is, of course, to pursue family reunion. However, in today's China, where population mobility has become the new normal, the action logic of a community group confined to a certain area could only be that different people come and go everyday. As a result, even those people who were actively involved in group activities no matter where they go, said, "Participating group activities is almost like staying in a hotel. You still don't feel at home."

Fourth, belonging only exists when there are homes to accept them. But the infected are also stratified. Among the backbone members of community groups, many have a relatively high status. As a result, the fact that they are all infected does not significantly reduce the gap between backbone members and the relatively lower classes.

However, these barriers are increasingly being broken by the logic of policy makers, health workers and infected people accordingly. Good policy makers try their best to provide convenience for community groups. Enthusiastic health care workers go to great pains to build "patients' homes". Infected people follow the principle that "something is better than nothing". Even if the result may not be satisfactory, many infected people gain a relatively strong sense of belonging.

(5) Revelation: gathering or being alone?

Two prerequisites for belonging: first, there must be an existing social unit which can accept them; second, both sides need to have strong homogeneity. But for HIV-infected people in China today, both conditions are lacking. Therefore, it is not surprising that some community groups are actually gathered according to their sexual orientation.

In my opinion, the so-called "HIV-infected group" is actually just a temporary collection driven by social discrimination. Even without talking about sexual orientation, there is also a great lack of homogeneity among people who are infected from different ways. During the, I have seen many times that some people with iatrogenic infection consider themselves innocent, so they often accuse those infected with drug abuse or sexual behaviors of being timid as a rabbit in protecting their rights, but they cannot understand the two latter's self-incriminating mentality—"reaping what one sows". Similarly, couples infected by sexual transmission urge people infected by homosexual behavior with persistence to "kick the habit".

The vision of regenerative home is actually the last choice, to find certainty for future life but in vain. But for those infected by sex or drug abuse, no matter how hard they and their partners try, they will find no ark to accommodate them in a short time, let alone the land of happiness.

Therefore, it's better to live on their own, learn to enjoy solitude and entertain themselves; at the same time, they also understand the meaning of a saying, "What you do not wish yourself, do not do unto others". They should learn to be independent citizens, striving for their rights and undertaking all responsibilities, yet willing to live on the margins of society. This is not an idiot's daydream. If you can see the increasing number of "homebody" and "single women" among young people, then that day will not be far away.

2.1.6 *Enlightenment from Research Perspective: The Co-Construction of Multiple Subjects*

The focus of this chapter: Not only does each party's own guiding beliefs and action logic constitute and construct each other, but among the policy executors, medical staff and infected persons, there is a more complex joint construction of multiple subjects too. This is not only a research perspective, but also a way to solve problems in the work practice: we should dispel blind worship and build a brilliant future by multiple subjects through improving the occasion in which the conflict of two sides exists.

This chapter is to cherish the memory of Mr. Li Hu, the infected grassroots activist. He is the full supporter and leader of the on which this chapter is based.

2.2 Infected People's Subjective Cognition of "Romance of the Three Kingdoms"

The aforementioned "Romance of the Three Kingdoms" is a concept that I summarized to describe the interaction and current situation of some organizations in the field of defending AIDS. That is to say: the Center for Disease Control and Prevention (hereinafter referred to as CDC), medical workers and volunteer groups, form the "Three Kingdoms". There should have been a cooperative relationship which can encourage them to move together between the three parties; but in real life, "the Three Kingdoms" often have some contradictions or even conflicts, which have been seen by AIDS patients, the party being served, and kept in the patients' minds. When I went to ask for information, they described these contradictions conflicts vividly, which formed the "Romance" that will be presented below.

The previous discussion on "the two-way conflict of action logic" is an abstract summary highly condensed, but it is by no means water without source. Its basis is the entire content of an in-depth social survey to be presented below.

However, the reason why I did this is not only for the purpose of showing that the words are "substantiated", but also for the consideration of these two methodological levels.

First of all, all survey conclusions come from the summary of the original materials. Therefore, it has become one of the ethical principles of social survey to present one's own survey content in detail for readers to judge.

Secondly, all survey conclusions are only researchers' own cognition, neither absolute truth nor exclusive definition. Therefore, what researchers hope most is that readers can draw new and different perception from original materials.

Therefore, the first part presented to readers is the result of questionnaire survey and quantitative analysis. The qualitative research of original materials are placed in the next third section.

2.2.1 How Can We Let Infected People Tell Their True Feelings?

(1) Which method can be used to disclose the truth to the utmost extent? period: April to June in 2013

Survey objects: HIV patients who live in Tianjin prefecture, also called carriers (hereinafter referred to as infected people).

methods: I use computer questionnaire survey method considering the particularity of respondents' identity, the sensitivity of themselves and the content of which involves their personal privacy and the condition of directly related parties (CDC, specialized hospitals and volunteer groups).

The computer survey method used in this research has the following advantages.

First, traditional paper questionnaires may make respondents hesitate. On the one hand, they worry that their personal privacy may be leaked and their answers may have an adverse effect on the future diagnosis and treatment on the other hand. Therefore, I let respondents answer in front of computers by themselves, without investigators looking the answering process.

Second, computer survey programs automatically encrypt all answers and data, so investigators cannot see the survey data, thereby reducing the worries of respondents.

Third, computer survey can also test the logic of questionnaires and respondents can choose to skip some questions. Such operations can prevent respondents from making some simple logical errors and increase the speed of answering.

Fourth, computer survey also avoid errors of data entry in the latter period. After directly being decoded, the data can be used for statistical analysis.

Form: This survey is conducted in the mode of random searching. It is rather difficult to find infected people because they are usually anonymous and secluded to a certain degree, so we cannot conduct random sampling surveys. Using the form of random searching in volunteer groups, we conduct one-to-one computer questionnaire surveys in a closed room after receiving the consent of infected people who come to volunteer groups for consultation and services. After the, we pay corresponding remuneration to show our gratitude.

Analytical method: This report uses STATA12.0 to conduct statistical analysis.

(2) What kind of infected persons are investigated?

About 234 valid questionnaires are collected during this. For 2,291 infected persons reported in Tianjin, such sample sizes fully meet the requirement for large samples. The lowest number of answers is 55 and the highest reaches 94 due to the differences between individual experiences. The average number is 72.

The basic information of samples: there are 226 men, accounting for 96.6% and 8 women. Among them, about 218 adults are under the age of 50, accounting for 93.2%. 159 persons' domicile places are in Tianjin, accounting for 67.9%, including 118 urban residents and 41 rural residents. 75 are from other cities, including 42 foreign urban residents and 33 foreign rural residents. The above data is almost the same with the overall distribution of infected persons in Tianjin, and can reflect the situation of infected persons in Tianjin to a certain extent.

In terms of age, the average of the total sample is 35.13 years old (the median is 34 and the standard deviation is 9.15). The youngest is 18 and the oldest is 67.

In terms of education level, about 4.7% of the samples have attended elementary school, 12.4% junior high school, 26.9% high school, 26.1% junior college, 28.6% university or above and 1.3% none of them.

In terms of work situation, about 78.2% are currently employed, 10.3% having previously worked but currently being unemployed. This shows that more than 88% of infected people have worked or are working, and those who have never worked before account for only a small percentage, about 11.5%.

In terms of the income of past 12 months, the average income of the sample is 3823 yuan (the median is 3000 yuan and the standard deviation is 5250.98). People without any income account for 8.1%.

In terms of the marital status, there are 44.4% of the infected who are unmarried and single, 6.8% unmarried and living with people of the same sex, 1.3% unmarried and living with the opposite sex, 34.6% in the first marriage and having a spouse, 1.7% remarried and having a spouse, 10.7% divorced and 0.4% widowed. The sum of all statistics does not reach 100% due to rounding off.

In terms of the length of residence, there are 3.9% of the infected living in Tianjin for less than one year, the same as those living for less than three years, 23.1% living for three to ten years and 69.2% living for more than ten years.

In terms of raising children, 63.3% of the infected have no children, 30.0% one and 6.7% more than one child.

In terms of supporting the elderly, 23.5% do not need to support them, while 14.5% need to support one, 43.6% support two and 18.4% support more than two.

All the 234 people in the sample have been diagnosed as infected. Although 103 people, accounting for 44.0%, have been diagnosed, they have not started taking medicine. 31 persons have taken medicine for less than one year, 45 persons for one to three years, 50 for more than 3 years and 5 being in other conditions, accounting respectively for 13.2%, 19.2%, 21.4% and 2.1%.

During the period of being diagnosed and being treated, infected people will receive more examination and be charged with more fees if it is their first time to take medicine. According to statistics, the average expenditure for HIV patients to take medicine was 17,037 yuan in the first month (the median was 5,000 yuan and the standard difference was 20,915.1). In 2012, the average cost was 6473 yuan (the median was 4000 yuan and the standard deviation was 6148.9). In 2012, the average total cost was 9,803 yuan for treating HIV (the median was 5,000 yuan and the standard deviation was 9782.9).

2.2.2 *Who Discriminates Against the Infected? What Has Been Discriminated Against?*

Discrimination and stigma are issues that HIV patients need to face throughout their lives. In the early years, there were debates over whether infected persons were innocent or not. Fortunately, these debates have disappeared in recent years. However, how are infected people being discriminated against? If we do not have a thorough understanding of this question, then our anti-discrimination work will be done with twice the effort.

(1) Who discriminates the infected most?

Considering about the social discrimination, 44.4% of infected people think that discrimination is serious. 20.1% think that discrimination is everywhere and 18.4% think that the discrimination is common but not that serious.

Another question on the questionnaire: Have you really encountered any kind of social discrimination? As a result, 21.4% of infected persons suffered from it and 69.7% actually not. Analyzing the time of being diagnosed, we find the number of people who have not suffered from social discrimination has increased year by year, from 50 to 75%, while the number of people who have not has decreased from 22.2 to 19.7% year by year ($P = 0.000$).

So, who is really discriminating against infected people? Those who have actually experienced discrimination in person believe that the discrimination mainly comes from medical institutions, followed by public opinions and government agencies. The most serious discrimination also comes from medical institutions.

Such situations show that the current stigma and discrimination against HIV patients can be said to be "hearing a lot but suffered a little", and the source of discrimination "mainly comes from the official but the folk a little."

(2) The route of infection is the most principal aspect of being discriminated.

This survey asks a question about how they are infected. As a result, 28.6% of the HIV patients choose not to answer this question, occupying the highest proportion of being refused to answer among all the survey questions. Then, the survey asks again: why are you unwilling to say your infectious route? As a result, the proportion pf choosing not to answer accounts the highest.

So do infected people know how they are infected? Among those who are willing to answer, 62.7% know clearly and 33.7% are uncertain but can guess how, only 3.6% are unaware. Then another question asked: which channels do you think can get people infected most likely? As a result, about 93.8% think the answer is unsafe sexual behavior, including 3 women.

This means that the infected not only know exactly how they are infected, but also the main reason for their discrimination. This is the reason why they are unwilling to answer those questions. This also shows that discrimination and stigma in society are actually coming from the fact that most of the infection channels are considered to be "filthy", so many people think the infected deserved it.

(3) In-depth thinking on discrimination

The current situation raises several important questions for the prevention and treatment of AIDS, so I have to say a few more words.

The first question is that who should determine whether there is discrimination or not.

At present, some well-intentioned people search for various discriminatory sentences or words from media in order to oppose discrimination against HIV patients. If they find such sentences or words, they would lift up their voice: how serious the discrimination is!

But, first of all, how much does the discrimination account for in media content? Is it common or rare? In particular, the influence of various media is widely divergent. Judgment of the overall situation will miss by a mile without regard of such "weighting factor".

Secondly, even if the discrimination really exists, does the infected, as the subject of being discriminated, feel it themselves? Do they really suffer from it? The survey find that most infected people think that the discrimination is very common, but they rarely encounter it. So, can we say the discrimination really exists?

The second question is that who is being discriminated against?

Some kind people said categorically that discrimination stigmatizes all infected persons indiscriminately. Unfortunately, this finds it not true. As mentioned earlier, most of the subjects in this survey are men, who were infected due to homosexual behaviors. The discrimination they feel and encounter is mainly from this special identity. In other words, we need careful analysis to figure out whether the discrimination is against all people living with AIDS or purely against gay men. We cannot generalize it.

On the contrary, the women in this survey are basically infected by men, so they rarely feel or truly encounter any kind of discrimination. In addition to this, there are many people in China who have been infected by blood selling or blood transfusion, but they do not think they have been discriminated against. Instead, they issue much stronger appeals and initiate more social activities precisely because they are innocent victims.

The third question is that why does discrimination work?

First of all, only when the infected are truly being discriminated can we can talk about the effect of discrimination.

Second, whether infected persons think it is a form of discrimination or not will directly strengthen or weaken the true role of discrimination. For example, health care workers usually wash their hands after touching a HIV person. Some infected people think this is discrimination, but many do not think that because medical staff should wash their hands after touching any patients.

Third, the psychological condition of infected persons will also strengthen or weaken the impact of discrimination on them. For example, many infected people participate in the specific work of preventing and treating AIDS as volunteers. First, they are often more sensitive to discrimination. Secondly, discrimination does not work on them.

The fourth question is that whose discrimination can cause the most mischief?

This survey reveals that it is from medical staff and CDC. The reason is very simple: No matter how serious the discrimination of public opinion is, the infected can escape from it if they choose not to listen or look, so it hardly cause major harm. However, after being diagnosed, the HIV patients generally fall into the abyss of despair, vulnerability and over-sensitivity. At this time, medical staff and CDC are like their life-saving straw, carrying the last ray of hope of them. If infected people are discriminated by these people, of course the harm is far more greater than any other discrimination.

2.2.3 *What Do Infected People Think of the CDC's Work?*

The Centers for Disease Control (CDC) plays a role of prevention, control and diagnosis in the work of preventing and treating AIDS. In terms of treating infected persons, CDC's role is mainly manifested in the following aspects:

It is responsible for organizing the epidemiological of newly discovered HIV infection cases, summarizing and analyzing relevant information, establishing personal files of infected persons and submitting these files to the superior departments concerned.

It takes charge of collecting, sorting out and analyzing the HIV preliminary screening results and confirming the testing results of laboratory. After finishing these jobs, CDC will report these conditions to the AIDS Prevention and Control Center of the Ministry of Health.

It is responsible for collecting, counting up, analyzing and summarizing the epidemic situation and relevant information; the CDC also needs to enact long-term prevention and control programs based on surveillance and epidemiological researches.

It is responsible for organizing the random inspection of AIDS voluntary counseling and testing institutions, providing technical support and guidance for treating AIDS and common opportunistic infections, as well as providing consultation and care for AIDS infected persons or patients.

It is responsible for the storage, distribution and deployment of antiviral drugs.

The above work must strictly abide by the national AIDS prevention and control laws and policies. It should implement various requirements in the national AIDS testing standards and undertake the task of HIV antibody identification and preliminary screening in Tianjin, and so on.

It can be said that the service work of CDC is indispensable for infected persons from the time of being diagnosed, to drug collection, follow-up, regular testing and care. We select several aspects that are closely related to infected persons to evaluate the work of CDC.

(1) What happened when the infected were diagnosed?

The first diagnostic criterion for an infected person is the positive HIV antibody, with relevant tests to confirm. The HIV antibody test can be completed by many institutions, such as professional hospitals, CDC, and some community organizations. Once the HIV virus is found to be positive, CDC would confirm the diagnosis and issue a diagnosis report.

The first time to detect the HIV antibody to be positive is of great significance to infected persons. According to the statistics of survey samples, the first time to confirm positive antibody was in 1998, only including 3 cases. By 2012, there were 68 cases. Before 2007(from 1998 to 2006), there were only 18 confirmed cases in Tianjin. From 2007 to 2010, about 30 cases were diagnosed each year, and 99 cases were diagnosed in 3 years. After 2011, 50 cases were diagnosed every year. From 2011 to 2012 alone, 117 people were diagnosed as infected in Tianjin, accounting for 50% of the total sample. Among 234 samples, 206 were diagnosed in Tianjin, accounting for 88%.

Many infected people did not participate in the first HIV test actively. Some infected people accidentally found their HIV antibody positive when they went to a general hospital. 48.5% were tested at CDC, 23.8% under the mobilization of the community and CDC, nearly a quarter of infected people at various hospitals, and 4.9% with test strips by themselves.

Through the analysis of the contingency table of the first HIV test and the time of being diagnosed, it was found that as early as 2007, the institutions for the first test were mainly distributed in CDC and hospitals, and less than 15% were tested under the mobilization of the community and CDC. However, from 2007 to 2010, CDC was the dominant institution for first testing, accounting for 73.3% of the total. Beginning from 2011, a three-part pattern of CDC, hospital system and mobilization of community and CDC has been formed, each accounting for 36.8%, 29.3%, 27.4%. The chi-square test result was significantly different ($P = 0.000$).

(2) During the first screening, do infected people need to tell their identity? Is the opposite side willing to inform the test result?

During the first screening, the policy requires verification of identity. However, this survey finds that only 50% of infected persons have identified themselves.

If we take 2007–2010 as the diagnosis time, we can find that the trend of identity verification is decreasing, from 71.4% before 2007 to 35.9% in 2011, showing a significant difference ($P = 0.000$). This shows that identity verification for the first screening is becoming more and more lenient, also signifying that there are more respects for the protection of infected persons' privacy.

33% of infected people told their true identity actively to doctors or CDC workers during the first screening and 67% did not.

After the initial screening, the number of infected people telling their true identities goes in a V shape, falling first and then rising, from 42.9 to 20.9% before 2007, and rising to 41.5% after 2010. The number of infected persons not telling their identities tends to rise first and then fall. This shows that without policy enforcement, the degree of trust of infected people towards testing organizations decreases first and increases after, showing a significant difference ($P = 0.008$).

68% of testing institutions inform infected people the first screening results and 32% not.

Before 2007, the notification rate of first screening results was 64% and it decreased to 41.5% from 2007 to 2010, but then increased to more than 90% after 2010, featuring a significant difference of decreasing first and increasing then ($P = 0.000$).

With regard to the methods of notification, there were only two methods, mobile phone notification (accounting 79%) and personal inquiry (accounting 21%) before 2007. Between 2007 and 2010, mobile phone notifications accounted 81% and personal inquiries accounted 13%. The method of informing through volunteer groups has experienced from scratch to 5%. After 2011, the condition went in the way of a tripod, including mobile phone notification (accounting 46%), active inquiry (accounting 29%) and volunteer groups notification (accounting 19%).

93% of infected people need one week to half a month to receive the testing results. 84% think that the first screening is unlikely to expose their identities. 15% think there is a little chance and only less than 2% (3 persons) think that their identities would be entirely exposed.

(3) Which party provides more guidance or consultation?

Guidance or consultation is indispensable for the diagnosis and treatment of HIV. Generally speaking, among the institutions that first provide guidance or consultation, 51% of infected people choose CDC, 31% volunteer groups and 14% hospitals.

Analyzing the time of being diagnosed, we could find that the number of people choosing CDC to have guidance or consultation tends to increase first and then decrease; on the contrary, the number of people choosing hospitals tends to decrease first and then increase. Only volunteer groups have more and more patients. After 2011, a psychological counseling model comes into existence, coordinated by volunteer groups (accounting 42% as the mainstay), CDC (accounting 35%) and hospitals (accounting 18%), showing a significant difference ($P = 0.000$).

So, what caused the change of first increasing and then decreasing in CDC's counseling or consulting work?

90% of infected people think CDC's attitude is relatively good. There are more people who think that CDC's attitude is particularly good and less people who think that it is relatively good. But the overall situation is stable, the recognition degree reaching around 90%. It can be seen that the service attitude does not affect the choice of infected people.

In terms of whether guidance and counseling are useful, 89.8% generally believe that they are useful. The difference is that the proportion of people who think that CDC's guidance and counseling are extremely useful is increasing year by year, and the proportion of people thinking relatively useful is decreasing year by year. We can see that the information provided by CDC is generally recognized by the infected.

From the above two aspects, we find that the number of infected people consulting in CDC first increases and then decreases, but the reason of such condition may not lie on CDC. On the one hand, CDC is also making further improvements in guidance or consulting. On the other hand, possibly it is the development of hospitals and organizations of infected persons that have brought changes to CDC. About this point, further analysis is needed.

(4) What about the detection of virus load?

In short, viral load testing measures the amount of HIV in each milliliter of blood. It is like the CD4 test, using a certain standard to measure the health conditions of the infected. If possible, infected people should be tested regularly for viral load. However, this survey finds that nearly 40% of infected people have never tested their viral load since they are diagnosed. 27.4% are tested regularly once a year.

Among infected people who are not regularly tested, 52% think that it takes money and they could not find an institution for free testing. 36% say that patients without taking drugs would not be tested. This ratio is also close to the ratio of infected people who have never undergone viral load testing. Therefore, hospitals and CDC still have much room for improvement when it comes to viral load testing.

In terms of the time to know the results of viral load tests, nearly 70% of infected people say that it takes one month, and only less than 10% can get the results within a week. It can be seen that the efficiency of virus load detection can be further improved.

(5) Why do infected people become increasingly dissatisfied with CDC?

Through analysis, we can find that the development of the CDC remained unchanged overall, but in the cognition of infected people, it is decreasing generally. The reason of this is not that CDC itself has gone backwards, but that the development of other institutions makes it backward. Especially the development of volunteer groups and hospitals, inevitably leads to a downward trend in the trust degree and satisfaction degree of infected people towards CDC.

But we have to say that CDC has a bottleneck on its development. In terms of providing assistance to the infected, CDC is obviously lagging behind volunteer groups; In terms of providing treatment to the infected, the expertise of CDC has been questioned compared to professional doctors. Therefore, it is worthwhile to further consider that what kind of role CDC should play in the "Romance of the Three Kingdoms" to better help and treat the infected.

2.2.4 How Do Infected People Evaluate the Work of Hospitals?

Generally speaking, hospitals are mainly responsible for establishing files for HIV patients, testing, prescribing drugs, providing treatment for opportunistic infections and other diseases for the infected.

(1) What happened when infected people took their medicines for the first time?

Not every confirmed person needs to take medication. In the early stage of being infected by HIV virus, drug treatment is generally not required (except for the window phase), only regular CD4+T lymphocyte count determination required. If the testing result of CD4+T lymphocyte is less than 350 units per milliliter of blood, then first-line anti-AIDS drug is a must.

The found that the earliest confirmed person was in 1998 but the infected person who took medicines firstly was in 2005 and the number was very small. If we took 2007 and 2010 as two point-in-time for taking medicines, dividing it into three parts, we can found that 3.1% took the medicines for the first time before 2007, 50.8% from 2007 to 2010 and 46.2% after 2010. But so far, 44.4% have not used anti-AIDS drugs.

After excluding those who were diagnosed but did not require medication, the found that 22.2% of the confirmed people were diagnosed before 2007 and also took medicines before 2007; 38.9% firstly took their medicines between 2007 and 2010; 11.1% after 2010 and 27.8% never. Among those who were diagnosed between 2007 and 2010, 59.6% took medicines between 2007 and 2010, 10.1% after 2010 and 30.3% never. Among those who were diagnosed after 2010, 41.0% took medication after 2010 and 58.9% have not taken medication until now.

(2) When infected people took medicines for the first time, which party informed them the most?

For institutions which informed infected people the first time that they needed to take medication, 69% were in CDC, 25% in volunteer groups, and 6% in hospitals. It can be seen from the first time to take medication, that patients who took medicines before 2007 were all informed by CDC. For those who took medicines between 2007 and 2010, 78% were notified by CDC. At the same time, the notifying work of volunteer groups increased a lot, rising to 14%. After 2010, the CDC notification rate continued to drop to 53% while the rate of volunteer groups increased to 37%, and the notification rate of hospitals also increased to 8%.

Among infected people who were told by CDC to take medicines, 93% consulted with CDC or guided by CDC before taking medicines. Among those who were told by hospitals to take medicines, 62.5% consulted or guided by hospitals before taking the medicines.

In general, infected people are satisfied with the consultation during the first medication. Among them, 22.5% were quite satisfied with CDC's consultation, 72.5% relatively satisfied, only 5% dissatisfied. But on the other hand, among infected people who consulted with hospitals, none of them were quite satisfied, 87.5% relatively satisfied. This means that hospitals' consultation for the first time to take medicines still needs to be improved.

(3) How about the physical examination before the initial prescription and the follow-up medication?

Before taking medicines the first time, 97% of infected people had undergone corresponding physical examination. Even if some individuals did not have a physical examination, the doctor would ask their condition.

However, 51% of the physical examination reports for the initial prescription were not given to the patients. Only 25% of the infected took their examination reports. After 2010, 88% got their medical reports, and only 12% did not get their medical reports, showing a significant difference ($P = 0.000$). This shows that hospitals have made great improvements in this field.

Judging from the follow-up medication compliance of the infected, the free drugs generally received are first-line anti-AIDS drugs. Infected people mainly take lamivudine (3TC), zidovudine (AZT) and tenofovir (TDF) medicines in Tianjin currently.

At present, most anti-AIDS drugs are taken in combination. In general, among infected people who take medicines, the proportion is relatively higher of those having the repetitive prescription and of those who do not know their prescription.

From the perspective of CD4 load after taking medicines, the effect of medicines is quite obvious. 67.7% of infected persons' CD4 are increasing and 25.4% do not change much, only 6.9% decreasing. Regarding the side effects of medications, 18.5% thought that the side effects are large. 58.5% thought they are not serious. 23.1% thought they are small. This means that great progress has been made in the treatment of infected persons with drugs.

(4) Taking medicines is not a trivial matter

From the time of being diagnosed, 60.5% of infected people receive medicines within one week, 19.4% within half a month, 14.7% within a month. In total, 94.6% receive their medicines within one month.

Specifically, before 2007, 75% of infected people could get medicines within a week and 25% could get medicines beyond a week but within half a month; between 2007 and 2010, 72% could get medicines within a week and the number decreased to 6% for those who could get medicines beyond a week but within half a month. And 15% could get their medicines beyond half a month but within a month. After 2010, the proportion for those receiving medicines within one week was reduced to 47% and for those who received medicines beyond one week but within half a month was increased to 33%. 15% could receive their medicines within one month. There is a significant difference ($P = 0.024$). This suggests that probably due to the policy, infected persons must first go to CDC to get the diagnosis report, and then go to the designated hospital to get medicines, which delays the first time to get their medicines.

By 2012, would infected people get their medicines on time? About 98.5% of the infected received their medicines on time (including relatively on time and exactly on time). Specific to each year, 25% of those who started taking medicines before 2007 were still unable to take medicines on time; more than 98% of those who started to take medicines between 2007 and 2010 could to get their medicines on time. After 2011, the percentage of taking medicines on time has increased to 100%, showing a significant increase ($P = 0.000$). This virtuous operation, on the one hand, is due to policy changes and attention of all sectors over the years, making a huge improvement in safeguarding drugs for infected people; on the other hand, infected people themselves are increasingly aware of the importance of drugs.

In terms of the time to take medicines, 52% come to take medicines at the prescribed time, 27% at any time, and 10% taking medicines by appointment or on weekends.

Furthermore, among infected people who started to take medicines after 2011, 45.8% took medicines at any time, in a relatively flexible way. Among those who started to take medicines between 2007 and 2010, 12.1% took medicines at any time. But people who started to take medicines before 2007 were unlikely to get medicines at any time. This was mainly because they had long been used to a fixed time set by hospitals. Therefore, among infected people who started to take medicines before 2007, 50% took their medicines in the prescribed time, but after 2010, it dropped to 35.6%. The proportion of those who made an appointment to take medicines or on weekends was 50% before 2007. Between 2007 and 2010, it was less than 21%. After 2010, it was less than 19%, with significant differences ($P = 0.000$). This shows that hospitals have added various ways to take medicines on the one hand, providing convenience for the infected; on the other hand, some infected people are still used to take medicines at prescribed time, which is not conducive to taking medicines in time. Thus, hospitals need to do more publicity and popularization work.

So are infected people satisfied with the time to take medicines? 52% think it is convenient (including very convenient and relatively convenient). 47% think it is not convenient or very inconvenient. Specific to different times to take medicines, 75% of the infected who started to take medicines before 2007 considered it convenient; only 31.8% of those who started to take medicines between 2007 and 2010 thought it convenient; the proportion raised to 74.6% among those who started to take medicines after 2010.

In terms of the place to get medicines, 34% think it is convenient and 64% think it is not. Specifically, the proportion was 50%, 13.6%, 54.2% respectively for those who started to take medicines before 2007, between 2007 and 2010, after 2010.

Generally speaking, in terms of the time to take medicines, the proportion of infected people who think it convenient is significantly higher than the proportion of those who think the place to take medicines is convenient. 30% think that both time and place are convenient, and 43% think that both time and place are inconvenient, showing a significant difference. ($P = 0.000$).

Among those who start to take medicines after 2011, 52% think that both the time and place are convenient, and 22% think that neither of them is convenient ($P =$

0.000); among those who started to take medicines from 2007 to 2010, 11% think that they are convenient, and 22% think they are inconvenient (P = 0.006).

There is another special phenomenon. With regard to the existing methods of taking medicines, the recognition of it is clearly higher among people who are diagnosed after 2010 than that of the previous, because the lowest overall evaluation towards time and place to take medicines is made by those who started to take medicines between 2007 and 2010. One reason is that people who were infected before 2010 are used to the old way of taking medicines and seeing a doctor, the other is the various obstacles they encountered or the stereotyped effects of policies. But it may also because they are more aware of national policies, so the need for maintaining legal rights, the requirement towards CDC and hospitals have also increased accordingly.

(5) Which has the better service attitude, CDC or hospitals?

Overall, 64% think that CDC's service attitude is better. 19% think that hospitals' is better. 8% think that both of their service attitude are good and 6% think that neither is good. Among them, 72% of infected people who were diagnosed earlier in 2007 believe that CDC is better and none of them like hospitals; 78% of those who were diagnosed from 2007 to 2010 think CDC is better and 7% think hospitals are better; 50% of those who are diagnosed after 2010 think CDC is better, and 32% think hospital is better (P = 0.000).

Divided by the time of taking medicines, 75% of people diagnosed earlier than 2007 think CDC is better, and none of them think hospitals are better; 83% of those diagnosed from 2007 to 2010 think CDC is better, and 5% think hospitals are better; 47% of those diagnosed after 2010 think CDC is better, and 25% think hospitals are (P = 0.001).

Although the proportions of the above two categories are different, the overall trends are similar and both exist significant differences. This shows that compared with hospitals, CDC has better service attitude in recent years, but the overall trend is declining. Although the satisfaction degree towards hospitals is relatively low, it is increasing year by year.

(6) How do the infected respond to other diseases?

Even if infected people have other diseases, they are often reluctant to go to hospitals. 92.3% said that they rarely went to hospitals, and only 2.6% often went to hospitals.

Most of them go to general hospitals and community hospitals, few to infectious disease hospitals. It shows that, for infected people, it is precisely not the so-called infectious disease hospitals, but ordinary hospitals, that can provide diagnosis and treatment for infected people.

When infected people go to hospital, more than 80% worry about meeting acquaintances and being questioned about their illness. The second is being refused to have an operation and the third is being asked to tested HIV. We can see that HIV infected people's anxiety about being discriminated far exceeds the worry about their disease.

Only 11.1% of infected people who go to hospital admit their infection actively. The other 88.9% choose to conceal it. Among them, 89% and 88% are worried about being refused to treat by hospitals and being exposed.

Among those who go to hospital to see other diseases, 7.6% are found to be HIV-infected. 90% of them said that something bad happened after they admitted their infection. 80% among them were refused to get treatment and 70% believed that the attitude of medical staff had deteriorated due to their infection.

(7) Why can hospitals catch up from behind?

On the surface, hospitals have not been recognized by the infected. However, after careful analysis, it can be found that infected persons actually "love hospitals and doctors more deeply, and give them more responsibility accordingly." Infected people love them because they are more professional and can provide better treatment; infected people blame them also because they are more professional. When infected people need help, there should be no misdiagnosis, over-examination, discrimination and refusal of treatment, and so on.

However, hospitals and doctors are continuously making positive changes. If dissatisfaction and lack of trust are the main comments of hospitals, this is basically a stereotype of people who were diagnosed before 2010. Conversely, among those diagnosed after 2010, the proportion of patients trusting hospitals and doctors is the highest.

From the statistical analysis, it is also found that after 2010, the praise towards hospitals and doctors by infected persons has shown a linear upward trend. This also shows that hospitals have more room for development in the "Romance of the Three Kingdoms". In the words of an infected person: As long as the doctor gives us an affirmative look, his love is meaningful.

2.2.5 *Volunteers' Service for Others and Themselves*

The volunteer groups mentioned in this book are mainly organizations that are actively initiated by infected people to provide services to people affected by AIDS. Its main work includes publicity and education, consultation and testing, treatment and care, psychological support, peer education, drug compliance education, etc. It is actively committed to promoting the development of medical policies in local region, striving to create a good medical treatment and living environment for the infected, improving the quality of life of the infected, minimizing the second generation transmission and constantly strengthening the team's own capacity building to contribute to the construction of a harmonious society.

The survey sample includes 5 volunteers (accounting 2.1%), 9 backbones (accounting 3.8%), 23 activists (accounting 9.8%), and 147 infected people (accounting 62.8%, including women) who have much contact with the volunteer team, 50 infected people (accounting 21.4%, among them 4 women) who have few contact with the volunteer team.

In terms of the frequency to take group activities, 9.4% have never participated. 59.4% have participated in less than 10 times, 17.5% in 10–20 times, 13.7% in more than 20 times.

(1) Are infected people satisfied with the help of volunteer groups?

In terms of infected people's satisfaction degree with the help of volunteer groups to gain knowledge about testing, treatment or any other aspects, 64.5% of infected people are helped and highly satisfied. 33.8% are relatively satisfied. 98.5% are satisfied in total, much higher than CDC and medical workers.

In terms of infected people's satisfaction degree with the psychological counseling provided by volunteer groups, 62.8% are helped and very satisfied. 35.5% are relatively satisfied. 98.3% are satisfied in total. This proportion is also much higher than that of CDC and medical workers.

With regard to any specific thing in life (such as finding a doctor, regulating interpersonal relationships, solving financial difficulties, etc.), infected people are also highly satisfied with the help of volunteer groups: 43.6% are helped and very satisfied. 39.3% are relatively satisfied. 82.9% are generally satisfied. However, CDC and hospitals have basically done nothing in this regard.

If the diagnosis time is divided into two phases: after 2007 and after 2010, we can see that the number of those who are greatly satisfied goes into a U shape in terms of the satisfaction degree with the help of volunteer groups to gain knowledge about testing, treatment or any other aspects. 72.2% were greatly satisfied before 2007, but this proportion dropped to 42.4% between 2007 and 2010, and then rose to 82.1% after 2010. The curve of being relatively satisfied is just the opposite, showing a trend of first rising and then falling, rising from 27.8% in 2007 to 54.6% in 2010, and then falling to 17.1% after 2010. The same trend also shows in the satisfaction towards volunteer groups' psychological counseling and their help in any specific thing in life. This shows that volunteer groups have also taken detours in the course of its historical development.

(2) Which party do infected people trust more?

A question on the survey: "Who would you trust more if volunteer groups provide you with different knowledge or information compared with CDC or hospitals?" The answer is that nearly 40% trust volunteer groups more. 26.1% trust hospitals more. 19.2% trust CDC more. 7.7% trust all the three parties.

Further analysis finds that if we divide people according to the time of being diagnosed, 50% of those diagnosed before 2007 are more likely to trust the volunteer team, 11% more likely to trust hospitals and CDC respectively and 22% more likely to trust all the three. Among those diagnosed between 2007 and 2010, the situation is similar: more than 50% trust volunteer groups, 12.7% CDC, 12.3% hospitals and 5.9% all the three. Among those diagnosed after 2010, the most striking change is that those who believe in hospitals account for the most, those who believe in volunteer groups the second but significantly lower, and those who believe in CDC the third ($P = 0.000$). This suggests that the longer infected people receive volunteer groups' service, the less they trust hospitals and CDC, and the more they trust volunteer teams.

On the one hand, it shows that the work of volunteer groups need a long period to show their sincerity. On the other hand, it is shows that the earlier an infected person is diagnosed, the more likely he or she is to have experienced some kind of obstacles or difficulties from CDC and hospitals.

But among the newly diagnosed cases (those diagnosed since 2010), 87.2% are more likely to trust hospitals. This may because they trust the professional authority more, or because the overall medical environment has changed, but also probably because the time and activities they share with volunteer groups are not enough.

Among them, those who have participated in volunteer group activities less than 20 times are more likely to trust hospitals than those who have participated in more or less activities. Those who do not participate in volunteer group activities or participate in more than 20 times are more likely to believe in volunteer groups ($P = 0.007$). Accordingly, it can be believed that moderate participation in volunteer group activities can help improve the trust towards hospitals, but if the number is too much, people will trust volunteer groups more.

Regarding to the variation trend, the number of taking volunteer group activities has a significant impact on which side infected people believing more. Specifically, those who participate in less than 10 times trust volunteer groups least and trust hospitals and CDC most. However, as the number increases, trust in volunteer groups gradually increases and trust in hospitals declines slightly, but not significantly, while trust in CDC plummets to zero.

In particular, which party will infected persons trust more when the knowledge and information given to them are inconsistent? 86% trust volunteer groups rather than hospitals. This raises a big question for the whole AIDS prevention cause: Is this a good or bad situation? Should it be encouraged or reversed? Actually, this is a basic question of cognitive methodology: Is the objective medical measurement or the self-experience of infected volunteers more beneficial for infected people? This has not been able to solve this problem, which needs further study by future generations.

(3) What do infected people gain from volunteer groups?

42.7% of infected people think that they increase their confidence and promote their mental health, ranking the first. 25.6% think they gain knowledge and information, ranking the second. 22.7% think they are fighting for their own rights, ranking the third.

Further analysis of the time being diagnosed shows that people who were diagnosed before 2007 think that the most important gain is to fight for their rights (accounting 27.8%) and to obtain knowledge and information (accounting 27.8%). People who were diagnosed between 2007 and 2010 also rate fighting for their rights (accounting 39.4%) and accessing to knowledge and information (accounting 32.3%) as the most important; among those diagnosed after 2010, 65.8% think the most important is to improve confidence and mental health and 19.7% think the most important is to obtain knowledge and information. The difference between the three infected groups is significant ($P = 0.000$). In other words, the work of volunteer groups must evolve with the intergenerational renewal of infected people.

(4) In the eyes of infected persons, what are the most important advantages of volunteer groups?

The top three advantages of volunteer groups: better attitude, more convenient and timely (accounting 91%), more considerate (accounting 89%), and easier to keep in touch for a long time (accounting 85%).

According to the rank of advantages, 41.0% think that convenient and timely is the most important advantage. 23.1% think volunteer groups are more considerate, and 16.2% think they have better attitudes.

For infected people diagnosed at different times, those diagnosed before 2007 think that being considerate is the most important. Those diagnosed between 2007 and 2010 think a better attitude is the most important. For those diagnosed after 2010, being convenient and timely are considered the most important ($P = 0.000$).

This suggests that volunteer groups should adhere to these three advantages as while as providing targeted services with different priorities.

(5) How are volunteers promoting the introduction of relevant policies and the participation of infected people?

The activities of volunteer groups can be explained from three aspects: microscopic view, medium view and macroscopic view. From the micro point of view, the activities aim to help infected individuals to solve problems of survival and life. From the medium perspective, the activities help to coordinate resources, such as hospitals, CDC and other community organizations, to provide better services for infected people. From a macro point of view, it mainly works to promote the development of policy. Of course, the participation and support of infected groups must permeate into three levels.

At present, Tianjin volunteer groups are promoting the introduction of some social policies for the infected. In terms of promoting the "subsistence allowance policy for HIV infected people or patients in Tianjin", 68% of infected people are willing to participate in some activities, and 17% can participate with all their strength.

In promoting the introduction of "remission policy for regular testing fee of AIDS patients in Tianjin," 68% of infected people are willing to participate in some activities and 19% would spare no effort.

In promoting "remission policy for opportunistic infection fee of AIDS patients in Tianjin", 67% are willing to participate in some activities and 19% would spare no effort.

It can be seen that to improve social policies, nearly one fifth of infected people are willing to participate with all their efforts. About two thirds are willing to participate in some activities, and only about 5% are unwilling to participate or can only participate in a few activities. The reasons for their reluctance are mainly as follows: on the macro level, they feel that these activities are unlikely to succeed; on the micro level, they do not have the time or they are physically sick, etc. So there's a lot of room for volunteer groups to make progress in these areas.

(6) Volunteer groups can do great things

Volunteer groups are the lubricant in the "Romance of The Three Kingdoms", and should also be the pillar of the "tripartite construction". Through data analysis, it can be found that in many aspects such as peer education, counseling and services, volunteer groups have natural advantages and are generally recognized by infected people. It can be said that the role of volunteer groups among the three parties is to hold CDC with one hand, and hospitals and doctors with another hand. In the face of infected people, volunteer groups devote themselves to help and serve them. This kind of help and service is comprehensive and ubiquitous. If what hospitals and CDC do is more about survivable service, using their professional knowledge and skills to ensure the healthy survival of the infected. Then volunteer groups should not only work with hospitals and CDC to focus on survival problems, but also focus more on their lives. What volunteer groups are doing is not only a rescue in the blood transfusion way, but also a hemopoiesis type of help. Volunteer groups should work from micro, medium and macro aspects. In the micro aspect, aiming survival problems of infected people, it should assist hospitals and CDC to help infected people solve their current difficulties. At the middle level, volunteer groups can coordinate the other parties' resources to help infected people solve various difficulties in life. On the macro level, volunteer groups can lead volunteers to actively participate in the fight for policies and the protection of rights and interests, so as to achieve better assistance and self-help.

2.3 The Prevention and Control of AIDS: From "The Tripartite Cooperation" to "The Trinity"

2.3.1 What Do We Want to Discuss?

The previous discussion in this book was only about "the tripartite cooperation", using the statistical results from the questionnaire survey. Its advantage was that it can reflect more wider and overall situations of the respondents to a certain extent. But it also had disadvantages that it was difficult to deeply understand the feelings, motivations, aspirations of the infected person and other situations that are hard to quantify. In particular, it's easy to dismember a living individual into pieces of data so that we can only know about the patients partly.

Therefore, this survey spent more time and energy on one-to-one qualitative interviews. We made the interviews to explore the needs of the three organizational forces involved in achieving "the trinity", the degree they have developed and their visions for the future.

The concept of "the trinity" was not put forward by the author, but an idea and slogan advocated by many infected people and volunteers all over the country since the beginning of the twenty-first century. It mainly means: volunteers, CDC and hospitals should be more closely united. Their joint force can serve the infected people, know their dilemma and needs better and move forward the whole fight against AIDS.

(1) A large variation between the infected people

Taking 2007 and 2010 as the cut-off point for diagnosis and drug taking, we can learn from the data that the infected persons diagnosed between 2007 and 2010 are mainly middle-aged people aged 30 to 39 years old, with senior high school education generally. The first-time marriage and single people were in the majority, and most of them had aged parents and young children. At the same time, in terms of income, their average wages are generally significantly higher; In terms of cost, they spent significantly more on medication and treatment both in the first month of taking medicine and in the whole year of 2012.

In addition to the significant differences in demographic characteristics, the patients diagnosed between 2007 and 2010 were highly satisfied with CDC and they had the closest relationship with CDC. Their diagnosis, counseling and consultation were mainly in CDC.

However, their satisfaction with the hospital was the lowest, regardless of the time, place or the way of taking medicine. In the service attitude of CDC and hospitals, more than three-quarters of them think CDC is good and only 7% think that hospitals are good. Hospitals are also at the bottom of the list in terms of the question which institutions they believe most.

In addition, those who were diagnosed from 2007 to 2010 paid more attention to fighting for their rights and interests. In contrast, patients diagnosed after 2010 believed more in hospitals and doctors; while those diagnosed before 2007 believed more in volunteer groups. Therefore, it is necessary to adopt different intervention methods to provide well-directed help for the infected patients diagnosed at different time.

(2) Infected people and "the tripartite cooperation"

Overall, the patients' satisfaction with the three parties is relatively high, but different infected individuals have significant differences. It is regularly shown that their satisfying or dissatisfying institutions with different diagnosis time are in the same. Although it is due to their different inclinations, this finding is a better confirmation that the unified and unitary treatment and intervention mode cannot solve the actual problems of different infected people.

In the face of a wide variety of infected people, CDC, hospitals and volunteer groups should cooperate with each other and develop in multiple ways. Only in this way can they maximize the intervention of infected people. From the data, we can find that there are many complements among the three, which precisely provide the corresponding help and services for different infected people. In other words, the treatment must break the previous situation of independent work, and call for the integration of the three. Therefore, the subjective and objective conditions for the transition from "the tripartite cooperation" to "the trinity" are mature. What needs to be further developed is how to coordinate development and realize the treatment service oriented to the infected.

2.3.2 How is "The Trinity" Progressing in Volunteers' View?

(1) Basically satisfied with the service provided by CDC

CDC was OK. They called the infected person regularly and had CD4 tests for them because they needed to be evaluated regularly. If they did not give the infected person CD4 test twice a year, the performance appraisal would be deducted.

Our cooperation with CDC has been many years since 2007. Not at the beginning, but now our cooperation is very good. If we still fight now, that is because we both have problems.

In fact, the director of X district was the one who has done the best job in finding infected people. He voluntarily went to places at high risk. You knew these high risk people, right? The researcher asked: like homosexuality? The volunteer answered yes. They would go to public baths and places like that, and they would go and find out who might be infected, and get them tested. Generally, infected people are willing to do these tests, because they are free of charge.

Take an example. I once volunteered for a infected man. And the CDC asked him how he was infected. The female doctor of CDC was particularly straight forward and she asked, are you 1 or 0? (1 stands for the top; 0 stands for the bottom.)This is the special symbol for the medical inquiry of MSM. The infected man was embarrassed. Think about it: he's a gay, and he's embarrassed when asked by a woman. Unlike us male volunteers, we did not care about that. On another occasion, we went to L bar for a test when the CDC brought in two interns from a medical university, a boy and a girl. The girl was born in the 1990s. She was very smart and lively. They got there to do an epidemiological survey that was to ask you what's going on. The girl was very calm and may be for the reason that she was a fujyoshi herself. It's particularly easy to accept this. She asked, "did your recent sex take a condom?" (Imitate a girl's voice) This guy was particularly shy. And the little girl said, "You had to be more protective of yourself, regardless of anal or oral sex." (Imitate a girl's voice with a laugh) The patient felt embarrassed. And it's actually a positive thing to do, because the people at CDC accept that. But the uncle thought, oh, she was a girl and younger than me, but more open than me. In fact, it needed to adapt gradually.

The confirmation of an infected person requires a report from the CDC. The real experiment has to be done by them. We volunteers are very responsible for the screening of abnormalities, but we can't say you are infected. Only the CDC has the authority to say, and the CDC has to do at least two tests. Both positive results means you're infected. We volunteers and CDC still have a lot of overlap in the process of getting the drug. But on the CDC side, they studied epidemiology and they learned how to control its spread not how to treat a disease.

(2) Conflicts of interest between volunteers and CDC

CDC had committed 20% of its money to our volunteers this year. We had to pay 5–8% taxes, and hire an accountant. Doing this kind of social work is supposed to be tax-exempt. There's only one way to get tax free, and that's to register as a nonprofit. Non-profit organizations have a potential condition, which is to have a higher competent unit. If you go to the CDC ask for help, you will compete with it for resources, which was what the CDC was concerned. We have worked for so many years. But I've only been paid for thirteen months from January 2012 until now. We originally planned to pay the salary on the 10th of every month, but now we can't get the salary until the 20th. I think in the process, I'm getting closer to the system to develop Social workers in China. But that's not something we're thinking about right now, because there's so much more to the fight against AIDS. Why would I want to do that? Because I am an infected person, I feel a sense of responsibility and a sense of crisis, I will fight for it, or wait for death.

We volunteers are not lack of strength, but simply don't have the opportunity to develop. In 2010, for example, we found that this was not the right way to do it, through CDC bidding. At the national level, 20 percent of the money is spent on tendering. But what we found was that bidding went wrong everywhere. When we did the research, we found that about 13 percent of the money was the volunteers applied for using. After we taxed, it will be only about 8%.

I was going to write a project for CDC bids, and then there's the competition on the project investment fee obtained from the tender. However, we can't see the money that the state put in, and also cannot see the money that the local governments put in. We worked with the CDC and sometimes we had conflicts, and the tendering system was the crux of the problem.

At the beginning, I didn't care so much, didn't care whether I was a volunteer because someone needs help. And then, as the work got more, we gave the CDC stipends, gave them specialist fees, and then reimburse them for travel expenses. Sometimes we felt unfair because we don't have enough money. But they said, "You are volunteers, you should be dedicatory." Ah! It's their work but they don't do and they ask us to do it for them. They'll get extra pay when they come out at night, and if their unit don't pay, they'll get it from us. They got a lot of money but they didn't do anything. And let us develop the spirit of selfless dedication. They thought that you volunteers shouldn't have subsidies, shouldn't have meals and shouldn't have anything.

We have these offices now, which we get all our money from projects to build. And what were the projects in the past? We are paid 62 yuan for a homosexual test, 300 yuan for caring for an infected person a year. The maximum allowance for a day's work today is 50 yuan, which we can submit an expense account from the project. They just let us do the work and paid little for us. Although I don't have the treatment of a social worker, I still think of myself as a social worker, not a volunteer, for the need of society. However, our country lags behind in this aspect and does not have a mechanism.

In reference to some foreign situations, the CDC should have some data, make some policy recommendations, and suggest about how much money should be spent. It is more effective for them to do so. We have to be cooperative because it used to be cross-cooperation. If we don't match well, what should we do if they make excuses like "the machines is broken, come back the next day"? Once an infected person needed to shift medical record. He used to live in Chongqing, but now he lives in Tianjin. It would be convenient for him to take medication and CD4 tests if he had his file transferred. If he was in Chongqing, it would be troublesome to go back once every three months.

The CDC does not do purely medical things. What the CDC wants is to raise the awareness of safe sexual behavior in these people. What they want is to meet the index. Even if you give them donkey's blood, they will test it for you. They don't take into account the needs of the infected. For example, the patient has just been diagnosed and the CD4 indext was 330 today. (It can be dangerous when the index reached 330.) They don't care whether your CD4 index dropped 3 years ago or it dropped just within 3 months. (If it's 3 months, the patient is in the acute phase and needs medication right now.) But they don't care.

In the long run, the CDC doesn't have a lot of technology and they don't make a big difference. Hospitals can do that, and the CDC can't replace the role of hospitals.

The people in CDC were all government officials, and we were all ordinary people. To be frank with you, this was a question of mentality. They didn't really understand that we NGO and CDC had a cooperative relationship. We organized mobilization and provide places. CDC only provided technical support, testing and blood sampling. We had a cooperative relationship, but their initial mentality was not good. They felt that they were government workers, so they were superior than your masses. There was some friction at first, and then it was all right. They gradually understood that volunteers were also hard-working for infected people's health.

(3) Praise of hospitals and doctors

In its earliest days in 2007, Tianjin's medical level was poor. It is also introduced by others that Beijing You'an Hospital is quite good. They also have a project, the 11th Five-Year Plan of the country. They asked if you were willing to join the program and get a free checkup. It's all free and good to me. Why don't we do it? So I kept checking. The 11th Five-Year Plan is followed by the 12th Five-year Plan. (The investigator asked if there would be more.) During the 11th Five-Year Plan period, I was given 200 yuan back to Beijing for a visit, but I didn't get paid during the 12th Five-year Plan period. But at least inspection fees were free. In fact, it didn't matter to me whether it cost more or less. It is mainly because the relationship has been established here since 2007, by taking physical examinations once every three months, such as CD4, viral load, etc. And it was good for you to continuously take medication, prevent side effects, and so on.

As for the hospitals, a Sunshine Medical Conference was held in Tianjin last year, which meant that they hoped the attitude of doctors could be better and better, even if you pretend to have a good attitude. We were coming for therapy and you had a bad attitude. (The investigator asked. How many people give you the cold shoulder now?) We met few doctors who gave us a hard look here. And the hospitals in Tianjin have improved much.

The cost in specialized hospitals was higher than others, of which Ditan Hospital was very good. I made very good personal friends with the head nurse of the Infectious Disease Hospital in Beijing You 'an Hospital. I asked the head nurse how to thank her. The head nurse said, "Don't thank me. Write us a thank-you note." I said ok. No problem. Then I wrote a thank-you note and sent it to the head nurse's mailbox. It's fine. Then after a day or two, the chief of staff of the hospital called back and asked, "How was the patient?" To be honest, the doctor really didn't have to come back and give you a call, just because we're on good terms.

I (the volunteer) prefer to introduce the infected person directly to the infectious disease hospital. He answered the phone as soon as he saw it was me. I told him, "We had a patient here in the inpatient department, and they asked us to go to Beijing." "There was no need to go to Beijing. Firstly, you should give him some medicine. Then took his temperature, and talked to the doctor about what injections to give." This was a very simple thing. That's something really troublesome to go to Beijing once have a fever. When we found this situation, we informed the hospital, reported the symptoms to them, and got a relatively independent outpatient service.

If you registered a specialist or a general doctor, you can't talk as long as we do. All you can say was that you had a cold and took some cold medicine after returning home. If he spent too much time with you, the next patient would be dissatisfied.

As long as the doctor was sincere to the patient, the patient would be satisfied. I can understand the clinicians, who were very tired. Just one or two doctors need to undertake the work of the whole city and they watch so many patients every day. So I understood that they may have a bad attitude. I said, you should put yourself in the other person's shoes, should you?

(4) Still many shortcomings in hospitals

The problem now is mainly discrimination in hospitals. There has always been discrimination, more or less. On the other hand, sometimes they didn't take the patient seriously, and the hospital service attitude was not good. The main reason is discrimination.

It's all free medicine in Tianjin. It should be free domestically, too. When using drugs, the doctor would try to make you use first-line drugs, which was a low cost. Now it's all free medicine. But those with medical insurance have to use medical insurance. Medical insurance is divided into three parts: outpatient, inpatient and medical treatment for serious diseases. We can't afford medical treatment for such a serious disease. So I asked, which step should we go to see the doctor? I had two or three thousand yuan in all. Taking outpatient service was not suitable apparently. If I was in hospital, the money would run out soon. If I was hospitalized for some other illness, I had to pay for it myself. I said wool came out of we sheep. It was useless to say that and it did not reflect the "four exemptions and one care". It's not that they intentionally skimp on us, but that they don't have a sense of it. So, in the trinity, I thought there should be further work, such as viral load and CD4 testing. And we patients who needn't take drugs didn't have to go to the hospital.

Now even hemorrhoid operation requires an HIV test. If you have HIV, they won't have hemorrhoid surgery for you. Last year, for example, a gay man suffered from anal abscess and condyloma acuminatum. He went to the K Anorectal Hospital. He paid 4,000 yuan for hospitalization fees and examination fees. Finally, he tested positive for HIV. The doctor rejected the diagnosis, charged the test fee, and refunded the other fees. (The investigator asked, did you think the hospital pursued any interests) Of course. All departments of the hospital are contracted or connected with each other. Even if they are not contracted, will hospitals pay doctors the same salary if obstetrics and gynecology made a profit of 100 thousand yuan for the hospital in January and orthopedics made 50 thousand yuan. Maybe everyone's salary is the same, but the bonus is different. Even if there is no contract, how to generate income for the hospital? Where does the money come from? They all come from patients. A disease that used to cost 200 turned 600. And the hospital returns the benefit to the department. It is something that we all know. Anyway, hospitals must have something that should be reformed.

In 2001, a waiter in our bar who was also infected, had a fever of more than 40 degrees for three consecutive days. At first we took care of him and took anti-inflammatory drugs for him and gave him anti-inflammatory injections. But the high fever didn't go down. At 12 o'clock in the evening, we drove him to the hospital. At that time, the big iron door of the AIDS inpatient department was closed with the room almost dark, where just a small light was on. We went to the special section for AIDS patients, which was in the infectious diseases hospital but quarantined. (There was no one in the AIDS inpatient department). Then we went to the lobby of the Infectious Diseases Hospital. We said to the doctor honestly, "This was an infected person with a high fever for several days. Please give him treatment." The doctor said, "We could't handle it. You had to go to the AIDS ward." I told him there's no one in the AIDS department and please contact them for me. Later, the hospital department called me. They said that you should go to Beijing when you had a fever. It was midnight and he asked us go to Beijing. So I picked up the phone and said, "Why are you talking like that? Go to Beijing just for a headache or fever? Wouldn't you have a headache? You can handle this fever. Why did you ask us go to Beijing? Where did you get this attitude?" The staff of the inpatient department said, "Oh, we have no one available here." "Click", then I put the phone down and talked with him no longer.

In the early days, there were contradictions between doctors and patients. It was because doctors discriminated against infected patients and they were indifferent to the patients. The hospital once had a director in the liver department. And the way of diagnosis and treatment was special. Many people came to take examination of liver disease and they were all around here. And there was no special AIDS examination room. If AIDS infected people went to see liver disease, they were asked to show the doctor their diagnosis report for the first time. An infected person would be afraid to be seen by others and would hand it to a doctor carefully. The doctor picked it up and said, "Ah! You are an AIDS patient. Are you gay or straight?" He said that when a room full of people were watching them!

Some infected people didn't ask us or other volunteers for help and they went to other NCDS hospitals. But the doctors didn't treat them carefully. Last year CCTV reported that a child who was suffering from cancer. He went to the hospital for an operation. But when he tested positive, the hospital turned him down. If the hospital had enough conditions and technology, I thought they shouldn't turn the patients down. Because the doctor knew the disease better than us. If they exclude us patients, it's against professional ethics. It's truly risky for them to operate. But as a doctor, they should know more about the ways and means of infection than us. And you had the ability to have operations. Do you still need us to help you?

(5) Volunteers' views on the trinity

(The investigators asked, he has heard that the CDC, hospitals and volunteers had different benefits and focused on different things. Thus, the cooperation between them was difficult. Why not let them restrict each other, like "the tripartite" political system. What do you think?).

Actually, I thought it was a good idea. But in China's current situation, it is not feasible. In China, the government had more power than society. What volunteers could represent was a small part of some groups. The other two are the superior side. As volunteers, how could they restrict the other two sides, the functional department of the government.

First of all, only if you have power in your hand, can you restrict them. Not necessarily actual power, but you should own leverage. Now, volunteers only have society and just these people as leverage. However, the hospital and the CDC thought, whether you had patients or not was none of their business. Even if you didn't have those people, I was still the section chief of the hospital.

If everyone could focus on the infected person, the problem would be much easier to solve. But now, each is pursuing its own interests, including some volunteer groups. For example, one day, the infectious disease hospital let volunteers in to set up a point-of-care, but they didn't pay the staff salary and any other costs. The volunteers would say, we did an extra job so there is an extra labour cost. But you didn't pay for us. How could we do it?

It was difficult to restrict each other's power. At least for volunteers, there was no power to limit others. Moreover, the CDC and the hospital had the superior-subordinate assessment system. So volunteers had no way to check others. If it really was a tripartite cooperation, tied together by some interest, it may breed corruption. They may think that since we can restrict each other, well, let's falsify together.

All the CDC gave us was technical support, like quarterly CD4 tests, providing CD4 indicators, or making annual viral load tests. The hospital was to examine the body, give you whichever medicine should be used and collect fees. The volunteer group was to do follow-up care, psychological treatment, emotional outpouring. Some little things that the patients didn't want to talk to the CDC and the hospital, they came to tell us. After all, we were the same kind of people as them. There was no barrier between us.

CDC supported us not funds but some daily supplies, such as some office supplies, printing paper, blood drawing tools and gloves. We also had our own project to support some things we can do on our own. Their support was limited because they needed approval from the superior. At the beginning, they provided the computer, but it was a long time ago, like 2007 or 2008.

We volunteers acted as bonds. Some infected people may not cooperate well with their doctors, and some may even be unwilling to face them. Our greatest function was acting as bonds between them. (The investigator asked, what was volunteers' relationship with the CDC in general?) When we did a global fund, we were going to be hosted at the CDC, which was to be affiliated. (The investigator asked, just attached to the CDC, get paid and you could do activities.) That's right. Then we did "the China-Gates Project", which was a cooperative project between the Chinese government and the Bill Gates Foundation in the field of AIDS prevention and treatment. The CDC would provide the doctor. We acted as bonds. We did what they couldn't do, vice versa.

CDC has been absolutely supportive in our work, and we've cooperated well. If we need supplies, they can give us. But when it came to money, there was a limit.

The difficulty of the realization of "the trinity" lied in discrimination.

Volunteers did not have enough unity for fame and wealth. Our team was on the side of the infected. There were gay groups, but we couldn't work with them. Let me give you an example. At the time of the bidding in 2010, in Tianjin, the situation was very complex. The CDC was supposed to give me a big cake, but they only gave me the horn of cake. I said, it is wrong to divide this way. They give too little. And we volunteers should fight for bigger interests. But the group was satisfied with 6 percent of the cake, and that group was satisfied with 3 percent of the cake. Eventually, the volunteer groups pulled out fighting.

(6) The lack of institutional guarantee in the current good situation

(Investigator asked you just said that the cooperation between your volunteer group and the hospital. This communication mechanism was good. And I wanted to ask how this mechanism was established. Was it created by personal charm, or an agreement between the two parties?).

It was established by the individual, absolutely. At the moment, it was individuals who were trying to cooperate, including hospitals for infectious diseases and some other hospitals. We also tried to solve the problem of high treatment cost in Tianjin, but we can only find some good individual doctors, such as Doctor XX from AAA Hospital. When he was on duty, patients came with our referral letters and could be treated at a very cheap price. But it may not be treated at a low price when you change to another doctor, even in the same department of the hospital.

(The investigator asked if the doctor recognized you or your volunteer organization.)

The doctor recognized the institution. However, the relationship was made up of individual volunteers and doctors. Many times, we had this relationship on our own by the influence of our organization and others by friends' introduction. For example, they would tell us Dr. X was very good. If you had patients you could introduce to him. Then we would communicate with this doctor, and we would build this relationship.

The future of our volunteers depended on whether the government had this purchase service. The government did approve the purchase of services, but the exact time and how to buy them was still unknown. The policy was being made, but we can't stop working. Every day we should do testing and psychological care, chatting with infected people. We cannot stop our work.

(7) The problems of the establishment of institutions

Now China's infectious disease hospitals, or designated hospitals for infected people, are rarely general hospitals. For example, the infected person only had hemorrhoids, and the infectious disease hospital cannot have an operation because there was no surgery. The Infectious Diseases Hospital in Tianjin used to be a large liver disease hospital. But later opened this infectious disease hospital. So the simplest hemorrhoid surgery cannot be done, because they did not have anorectal surgery. At this time, you can only go to other hospitals.

There were even many infected people found in the hospital. He was operated on in other hospitals. He didn't know that he was infected until the physical examination before the operation. At this time, this hospital put the patients in the CDC and let the CDC do the diagnosis.

(The investigator asked, what about being diagnosed by CDC? If he came to the general hospital again, would they give treatment?).

That depends. For example, last year teacher X performed the operation on the infected person because it was really difficult to perform the operation on the infected person outside. Therefore, I hoped that this trinity hospital did not only refer to infectious disease hospitals. But at present, many infectious disease hospitals in China are not general hospitals. If you want to change them into general hospitals, it will require a lot of expenses and a long time, which is not realistic. Since there were available general hospitals, why can't we sort out a respective channel for infected people? And in fact, for medical staff, there was no additional risk of performing an operation on an infected person as long as they followed their occupational protection measures.

(The investigator asked, but these problems now are why general hospitals do not want to accept infected people?).

In fact, they would try to refuse them for all kinds of reasons. For example, if the infected person had any accident, we didn't have any methods to solve it here.

(8) Feasible advice: community groups enter the hospital

I thought at least we could take the first step. The volunteer group can be stationed in the hospital. In this way, more problems may be discovered in time. In many cases, patients only talk to our volunteers about the problems they encountered. At the same time, volunteers in the hospital can go directly to serve those who are more in need of services. For example, many patients who were hospitalized in infectious disease hospitals are in the hospital alone with their families not knowing and the medical staff may be too busy to take care of them. At this time, volunteers can help them well. At least we can do clinical nursing for the patients. In addition, the nurses are basically women. Some male infected persons had undergone some operations with a relatively weak body, making it difficult for them to get up to the toilet. If there were some volunteer companions, it could be handled well.

Our volunteers communicated very well with the medical staff, like the new doctor who came to Tianjin Infectious Disease Hospital, and their head nurse. If they have any questions, they will communicate with us at any time to seek our help. But it is impossible to move into another organization to work.

As we all know, the concept of volunteers is still very sensitive in China, especially Tianjin, which is a relatively conservative city. Therefore, the hospital does not dare to let the volunteers in, or they would have some concerns after volunteers entered. The hospital leaders think that even if the volunteers are not allowed in now, the condition of this hospital would not get worse. Because the hospital does not dare to predict what the volunteers would be like when they come. If it is good, it is certainly okay. What if it's worse?

For example, will the volunteers do something in the name of the hospital or else? At the same time, the hospital may also consider whether I need to give volunteers money, whether they need to give them a special venue. These may be things that the hospital should consider.

(9) More communication and getting closer

I thought that "the trinity" may also be a way to learn more about each other. Just like our current cooperation with CDC, CDC felt that volunteers were really helpful. If there are 10 people, they can only find 2 infected by themselves; but if we help CDC find them together, we may find 9 people for them. They saw the results of our volunteers' work.

However, we have done more extra work and the hospital cannot see it. For example, many infected people dare not take the medicine when it is time to take it. They may feel that once they start, they will take it for a lifetime. They need to take the medicine regularly every day. They will have more psychological burdens to go to hospital and use medical insurance. And they would be worried about being discovered by others by relatives. Those who were infected will have these concerns. The hospital couldn't see we helped them dispel these concerns. What the hospital saw was that one after another died.

To be honest, the hospital did not need referrals from our volunteers. When hospitals open, it doesn't matter to them whether you come or not. Of course, if more infected people come, the hospital's efficiency will be better. But you know, after the hospital's benefits are improved, the hospital's other costs will rise. For example, the hospital must forcibly test the infected person for syphilis. The hospital could have saved 80 yuan, but the policy stipulates that the hospital must do it once. This is also quite a contradiction for the hospital.

There is a Red Ribbon Home in Beijing Ditan Hospital. It cannot be said that volunteers are stationed in the hospital, but the hospital has established a non-profit social organization. I think this method is also very good. Because infected people have to go through going to the hospital. To be honest, this is inevitable. The infected person must be diagnosed by the CDC, and sooner or later they will deal with the hospital. Especially after being infected, it was very difficult to perform even some normal operations.

2.3.3 *CDC's View of "The Trinity"*

(1) Successful cooperation with the hospital

Our CDC had a lot of cooperation with hospitals. In the past, we had to supervise hospitals above level 2 every quarter, but now we have to do it every six months. The cooperation was mainly with the epidemic department of the hospital, and the outpatient service was mainly to contact the STD clinic. Although it was said that there was no distinction between sexual and AIDS, STD reporting was mainly managed here by the CDC.

The cooperation over the past few years has been very good. For example, when it is necessary to arrange tasks, I will talk about it when supervising. We hold a one-time HIV/AIDS testing meeting at the end of each year, at which we will talk about any tasks that need to be arranged. But there were some high-level hospitals that we did not have power to manage. This depended on our personal relationship. We had a good personal relationship with these hospitals, so we arranged the task easily.

At present, the municipal CDC and general hospital in Tianjin cooperated together. Tanggu approved a laboratory for diagnosis in 2010, and the others need to be sent to the diagnosis laboratory for confirmation. We were also afraid of the loss of information, so we will train medical institutions every year. If the patients are found to be suspicious in the initial screening, the second blood collection must be confirmed by telephone. We have to browse the preliminary screening information network every day. If the results are positive, we have to go to the hospital to carry out epidemiological, and then report the epidemic situation. We will take over the management guidance in the later stage.

Hospitals had to report data every month since 2005, and we needed to audit them. If there were infected people, we needed to report by phone, collect personal information, take blood and send it to downtown for a diagnosis test.

The work to dispense medicine was given to the hospital. Our CDC's job was a little easier than before. In fact, as far as the common people were concerned, when they went to the hospital to see a doctor, why did they have to go to CDC to get medicine? Infectious disease hospitals had procedures for medical treatment. CDC did not have clinicians, so the clinical problems of patients cannot be solved.

The cooperation between CDC and the hospital is now pre-operative testing. Because now the hospital will do a preliminary HIV screening before surgery, and it is relatively large work to do that. They also found many infected people every year. After they find out, we will conduct epidemiological s. They also have a preliminary screening laboratory. Usually after screening, the blood will be sent to municipal CDC for diagnosis. We can also go to collect blood, generally the faster one does it.

Who will do this work? Theoretically, it should be the hospital, because they found it. But our CDC can also do that. As the guidance agency of the hospital, we are more professional than the hospital. If there is not enough time, or if there are difficulties, we will also help the hospital in the epidemiological. There are many cases as such. Doctor X and I often go there. As long as the hospital is in our district, we have the responsibility to help them.

Since June 2017, patients have no longer received medicines from our CDC. They went to the hospital to collect them instead. In the past, the examination was done at the infectious disease hospital first, and then the doctor prescribed the prescription, and finally came to CDC to get the medicine after the prescription. But this process was very inconvenient for patients. Other cities have already sent medicine to hospitals, but it is not that in Tianjin. It didn't improve until 2017. In fact, we were very grateful for this policy, because the time for patients to collect medicine was not fixed and our work was relatively busy.

(2) Some remaining difficulties in cooperation

At present, Tianjin has designated only one infectious disease hospital. In recent years, our CDC has taken on too heavy tasks. With so many patients in 18 districts of Tianjin, some clinical case-based infections have occurred, which need to be treated in infectious disease hospitals. We transferred the information of patients taking medicine previously managed to infectious disease hospitals from May 24 to May 25, 2015. According to feedback from patients taking medicine in the past few years, it is true that the task of infectious disease hospitals is very heavy. All patients are concentrated there for half a day in the morning, and doctors cannot solve them one by one. We can understand that some patients have a big bone to pick with infectious disease hospitals. It's better now. Patients took drugs from CDC until the May of 2015, turning to the hospitals. We CDC were not only to give medicine, but also to solve patients' complaints, trying to make patients calm down. Actually, if there are too many patients, it's a little difficult for clinicians to handle and it is impossible for two doctors to solve all the problem.

Although the hospital is managed by the Health Bureau, the specific work is still undertaken by the CDC. We will submit the work plan to the Health Bureau every year and issue it in the form of a document by the Health Bureau. Of course, our CDC's work plan is also formulated based on the city's work menu and the actual situation in our district. I think it is necessary to consider infectious diseases more comprehensively, and it will be logical to implement them over time. If you add the plan little by little, the clinical doctor will not get used to it. If you think about it comprehensively at the beginning, it may be difficult to realize it at first, but it will become a habit after a long time.

Discrimination against patients was still widespread. In theory, doctors should treat patients equally, but doctors are also human, and they will also be afraid and try not to contact infected people. In fact, our CDC usually told doctors about the transmission route of AIDS, but they are afraid, because doctors often encounter wound problems during surgery, such as cuts, or blood splattered. But for people with AIDS, there are no special requirements for surgery. That is, how to protect people with general surgery and how to protect people with AIDS is enough. If you don't cut your hands, it's okay. Even if blood is splashed on your hands, it's okay if you don't cut your hands. In fact, there are still many ways of protection.

Now our district, including the entire Tianjin city, is a low-endemic area. The detection of HIV-positive cases is very limited, and ordinary hospitals do not have much contact with infected people. And when our CDC went down to publicize, we also asked hospitals to create a non-discriminatory atmosphere. We always told doctors this way, but after we finished talking about it, it's hard to say how far they can understand. The care follow-up is mainly done by the CDC, and the hospital has done very little in this regard, almost nothing.

(3) CDC are not managers but friends with volunteers

In the past few years, we CDC cooperated with community groups to intervene in the work and set off. In order to do a good job, we also recruit volunteers on this site because sometimes we are really too busy.

The community group has also undertaken international projects in recent years, like the Haihe Star Community Volunteer Group, the Deep Blue Community Group, and a caring community group, including our supervision and management working group, and the earliest community group for prostitutes. Well, whether we undertake national projects, do intervention and publicity work, we provide some cooperation. If technical guidance is needed, we will provide it. For example, when we go to some places for blood collection on Saturdays and Sundays, we will provide people with on-site consultations and answers. We are the relationship of cooperation.

It is more convenient for community volunteer groups to do some work than us. They are relatively familiar with the "gay" (homosexual) people and they are more convenient to contact. If the staff of CDC go to places where some "gays" gather, they may have some guard. If there are any questions about the volunteers' early publicity work, we will answer them, or provide blood collection services. In the later period, the "gays" gradually understood our CDC, as a government department, emphasized the confidentiality of information. After all, there will be some discrimination against this disease in the Chinese public. He recognizes you and will come one after another. Some people came to CDC last time and sat for a long time. You give him an answer to this knowledge, but he is indeed under a lot of psychological pressure and even has some psychological problems.

The relationship between we CDC with volunteer organizations was okay. The "China-Gates Program" required grassroots organizations to participate. The first was a joint project, the "Global Fund Sixth Round". Our CDC cooperated with volunteers to organize blood tests and went to them to promote AIDS related knowledge. The cooperation was good.

We CDC and volunteers had basically no conflicts or poor cooperation. We are still very happy to cooperate, but sometimes we need to negotiate on working hours. Like the intervention of prostitutes, we usually go at noon when they just get up or at night before their opening. It usually takes up our spare time, but we are okay with that. To work for people living with AIDS has to sacrifice personal time, because their work and rest time is different from that of ordinary people. It was better to manage when medicine was available before. They went to us to have tests and get medicine, and there was no conflict.

Our district CDC cooperates with the volunteer group. The volunteer group will be sent to the district with which the volunteer group cooperates. Generally, volunteers are rarely sent to the city CDC. Consultants prefer to go to municipal CDC.

The relationship between our district CDC staff and the volunteer team has been good in recent years, whether it is "Deep Blue" or "Haihe Star". In particular, "Haihe Star" is located in our district. Personally speaking, it cooperates well with them. For example, some friends were referred and tested positive. The mobility of these people is quite strong. Some people can't be found after they hang up the phone. I will find people in the community group to let them pay attention. Sometimes community groups will get together to chat, just find someone and ask him to contact me. We cooperate very well.

(4) Supporting "the trinity", but without satisfaction with the present situation

I always talk about "the trinity", which is also the advanced experience of other countries. In other words, the advanced experience was introduced to us, and the health department may refer to it in the future. I think it is quite necessary. In terms of AIDS prevention and treatment, it should be the government's initiative, the participation of various departments, and the participation of the whole society. In fact, I also want to write a paper. I want to understand what the "China-Gates Project" has on positive findings in our district, but I have never written a sociological paper, nor have I studied it. And I don't think it is appropriate to use statistics alone.

In the present, "the trinity" is only 60 percent done. I think the connection should be closer. "The trinity" is not yet in one at all. I think that in the future, there should be a process from positive discovery to "fluid regulation" follow-up to CD4 detection to referral to the organization of infected persons. Maybe Tianjin is a low-prevalence area of AIDS, so it has not yet formed a scale, like Guangxi is relatively large, and seems to be relatively mature.

The situation in this area should not be very good. This is related to the fact that Tianjin is a low-endemic area and has not attracted the attention of the government. In some high-incidence areas, such as Guangxi, Sichuan, and Henan, the government departments there will attach great importance to it, and the government will promote work if it attaches importance to it. There are definitely fewer refusals in high-incidence areas. The doctors see more, and there are many infected people, so if you don't treat him, no one will.

(5) The need for policy support

The hospital is responsible for the treatment. Community volunteers are mainly responsible for psychological care. In fact, we still need the help of the community group. Now the question lies in how we can cooperate in the future and how to solve the funding problems. It will be difficult if we don't have funds. The solution to the problem mainly depends on the country's supporting investment. Even if a policy comes out, the implementation of the policy will still take a certain amount of time, and it is even more difficult to allocate from top to bottom.

I think it should be coordinated by the government to set volunteer group in the hospital. I also heard some patients talk about other provinces and cities, such as

Beijing You'an Hospital, which set up volunteer groups to save patients from running back and forth. The message I got from the doctor is to communicate well with the community group. I think that this model is quite good, but Tianjin doesn't seem to have one yet. There is a caring community group, which seems to be in an infectious disease hospital. I am not very clear about it. The community volunteer group is best coordinated by the government. To put it bluntly, it will be beneficial for the country to formulate economic support policies in the future. This is my personal opinion. The government will take the lead, operate and integrate it through caring funds to make things better.

I think government departments still need to coordinate. The municiple CDC can't manage some relatively large hospitals, not to mention the CDC of the district. Some policies should be introduced by the government, which will be better. It is not enough to merely suggest that we do it. If there is no policy at the government, the health sector also can't do it.

(6) The need for objective conditions

Volunteers mentioned that they want to have an office in the CDC or hospital as an activity point. They can help maintain order, and they can gather and explain knowledge one or two days a week. I think it should be possible, but this has to be exchanged with the infectious disease hospital and the Tianjin health department has to build a platform. Because the workload of clinicians is too heavy, patients want to talk to the doctor more when they go to hospital, but the doctor may not be able to explain more. Therefore, I think this platform is very good and beneficial to the infected.

But at present, our district CDC does not have this condition. We will move to a new office building in the future. It is said that the office conditions may be worse. The health department, epidemic prevention station, supervision office, maternity and child hospital are all together. We sometimes think about staying in the old building instead of going there and working with various departments. Because the houses are full, there are no such conditions now.

But this kind of cooperation was still good, relying on each other's advantages. However, there was also a prerequisite, which was to ask for their consent. As far as I am concerned, some of the infected people and patients we found were referred to by community groups through publicity activities for testing, and some were diagnosed by medical institutions, outpatient clinics or activities, and we need to seek the consent of them. Our job is the equivalent of half a psychologist. Sometimes you have to understand his basic situation, do tests, and pay attention to his psychological changes. Some infected friends often would not talk to others and they would come to talk to you. But what should they do in the future?

The Binhai Community Group and the Deep Blue Community Group had caring groups for infected people and patients. They would help patients and solve their problems like a friend, listening to them, and providing them with help. We had their referral card here.

(7) The unpredictable prospects

It is impossible and difficult for the three parties to coordinate by themselves. Because the CDC and the hospital are at the same level. Even if we ask the hospital to do anything, it needs the superior to consent. If the superior does not have a policy, we cannot ask the hospital to cooperate with us. Our district is okay. For example, there are so many large hospitals in the Heping District, which are not under the management of Heping District CDC at all, and coordination is impossible. Those big hospitals don't even take care of the city's CDC. They are busy taking care of the patients. And they have no conditions. But working with grassroots organizations will be easier. At least there must be policy support before it can be done.

I thought the CDC played a great role in "the Trinity". The infected people were usually found in the hospitals. But the report, the circulation and the follow-up care after the discovery were all done by our CDC, and we are also doing all the subsequent referral services. In recent years, 80% of the infected men were gay. Every year only one or two prostitutes were tested positive while forty to fifty gays would be tested positive for AIDS. In addition, gay organizations had project support, and male infected people were more willing to find organizations. For one reason, they had the same sexual orientation. For another, they needed organizational care and the volunteer group had also done a lot of work. However, they still had to come to CDC to do regular tests. And CDC played a key role in doing the task. We also hope that more organizations can help us shoulder some of the work.

Compared with hospitals, our CDC had more contact with volunteer groups. The community group will manage many patients, and it will also create files to care for the infected. If the patient has many problems, the team can directly contact the hospital. Now the city is paying more attention to it, and it is also improving the issue of fixed medical treatment, that is, where should an infected person go to if he has an operation. Because some hospitals do not have the ability to perform difficult operations, I don't know if I have decided which hospital to do it now, but I will definitely do it in the future. AIDS complications will continue to increase. In many cases, many of the needs of infected people are not met.

Our CDC usually has quite big workloads! What I told you just now is just the tip of the iceberg. Those are just some of the jobs, and there are many other jobs. It is also responsible for the management of venereal diseases, such as syphilis. We have to report once a year. The work of each department of our CDC is in a relatively saturated state. That is to say, there is a huge shortage of staff. I really hope that more new people can join in our CDC.

We have also tried recruiting volunteers or interns. In the past, we had project funding, that is, the "China-Gates Project", but the volunteer group did not have funding, so we would cooperate with them. A few of us alone cannot accomplish these tasks.

In "the Trinity", the first consideration is regional issues, because it will be more convenient to work closer. Then pay attention to the previous cooperation. If the previous cooperation is pleasant, of course it will be given priority. Due to the relatively large workload in our district, we used to cooperate with four volunteer groups.

The number of gay blood collections was more than 4,500, which reached its peak. Or let them go to the work site with us to collect blood. If they are too busy, the volunteers will collect blood first, and then we will send a doctor to the scene to collect the collected blood, and finally do detection.

2.3.4 *The Hospital's View of "The Trinity"*

(1) Cooperation between the hospital and CDC

It is indeed impossible to let the hospital take over the AIDS patients now. This has to be negotiated between the government and the medical institution. I think the situation in our district is still good. If medical institutions find HIV-positive people, most of the infected people are clinical inpatients. Few of them are sent to STD clinics and VCT voluntary testing consultation clinics, which I think our hospital has done a good job. My requirement is to treat every infected person as a potential patient for protection, and there will be nothing bad happening.

Our hospital is the only one in Tianjin that is responsible for AIDS treatment. The prevention and treatment of AIDS has also received strong support from our leaders. The hospital attaches great importance to AIDS and has invested a lot. Recently, we have sent a doctor to study abroad.

In fact, our hospital has invested a lot in this area, and the leaders also paid great attention to it. The investment in the allocation of medical facilities and medical staff is very large. We also attach great importance to cultivating young newcomers, like our department Doctor Gao, who will soon go to Beijing to study. In fact, we lose money for every patient we receive. It is not like some people say that we make a profit from AIDS treatment. This is absolutely impossible.

(The investigator asked if the hospital still loses money for treating AIDS patients.)

The answer is yes. The state did not give us funds, and the hospital had to subsidize it. The doctors and nurses in our department have relative high bonuses, which are indeed all subsidized by ourselves. The hospital does not make a profit from the treatment of AIDS. In fact, we have done a lot of things, like the patient's information. I personally do each of them. We actually do many things, but we are too busy with our work. We don't have time to summarize it in time to the height of theory. We also want to cooperate with your investigators to ask for help.

Some patients had doubts. For example, they were afraid that they were false positives. So they asked if they could also get a diagnosis in the hospital so that they didn't have to run both ends? In fact, hospitalized patients will not go to CDC. Some patients who went to CDC were not seriously ill, and they were discharged before the initial screening results came back. That's why we require the hospital to collect personal information for the first screening. I am afraid that the patient will be lost. We should collect the patient's phone number during the first screening, in case it can't be found when the screening is required.

(The investigator asked if there was any overlapping work between the hospital and the CDC.)

There is no overlapping work. There are two different systems. The original CDC was in charge of filling out the form, and now it has been transferred to the hospital, which is equivalent to a one-stop service. However, the detection of viral load and CD4, and the diagnosis is still done by CDC, and the hospital does not have funding for this project. The medicine used to be taken at the CDC, but now it is taken at the hospital. Therefore, the problem of transportation expenses raised by patients before is no longer a problem. Now the patient has to go to the CDC 4 times a year, oh, 4 times in the first year, and 2 times a year later. In fact, it should be 4 times, but the CDC now only gives you 2 times. If you want to do the rest, you have to pay for it.

(2) Cooperation between the hospital and the volunteer group

Our relationship is very good. As you have just seen, we are very familiar with the volunteers, and we usually get along like friends. They come to us if they have any medical problems, and we are very enthusiastic to help them. And we would also turn to volunteer groups for help if we met patients who didn't cooperate. Our relationship is very good.

When someone knows that they are infected with HIV or that they have children or lovers, they will be extremely stressed. We will give them some psychological counseling to relieve their psychological pressure. Sometimes we will introduce these infected people to volunteer groups, and ask them to participate in some related activities. Their mood will gradually be better.

In fact, some patients are not serious, judging from their examination indicators. But their psychological pressure is particularly high. Even more serious appearing anxiety and depression, and they feel that they will be able to live within a few days. This situation may exacerbate the disease. So we have to give some psychological counseling to the infected person after telling them. I think the most important thing is communication to express the worries clearly. There are many infected people who do not understand and do not know the situation. So we have to tell these infected people some specific matters about the infection. Then, we will introduce these infected people to groups, which we have a meeting with today, such as the Haihe Star. Groups have some natural advantages. They can go deeper into the lives of these infected people and have a better understanding of their lives. It can allow these infected people to participate in some group activities to relieve their pressure. This will also benefit their illness.

In fact, community groups often take these infected people to participate in some community activities, and the leaders of these groups will often bring some infected people to our place for inspection and treatment. Because some infected people just learned of the disease. They may be in a rush and muddle, and don't know what to do in the hospital. The team leader is more familiar with the hospital and they will also lead them and help them.

(The investigator asked if the other two parties had any needs for the work of the hospital.)

There is a demand. We are not very easy to say about this. They will directly submit any requests to the health department, and the health department will notify us again. We are not a system, so they will not directly ask us if they have problems.

There is no direct communication between the three parties. As long as the problems raised by the volunteer team are reasonable, we will consult the superiors and then solve them.

2.3.5 Key to Solidarity: Interests in Coordination

The qualitative interviews demonstrate that the hospital, CDC and the volunteer group have the same fundamental interests of AIDS prevention and treatment. However, they may not coordinate well in cases of conflicting interests.

To start with, the volunteer group works in the front line, responsible for numerous time-consuming chores. It naturally requires finance with a high frequency. Nevertheless, despite hospital's and CDC's great supports for the group's temporary work, they still lack the money for their organizational development and daily management. Besides, the international fund, presently the mainstay of the groups, is factually eggshells for them to keep walking on, because the fund, in the single form of project, will get cut off as soon as the project is completed. That is why the groups are asking the national and local government to make their funds normal, daily, long-term and fixed. Although the "government purchase service" mode is making huge progress now, yet it still can not meet the actual needs of the group.

(1) Community groups' concern on this issue

Such cooperation calls for the distribution of resources for which groups may quarrel: I can do the job, but how shall we share the money? Something like that.

Also, there will be conflicts between the hospital and CDC - I mean, some intrinsic contradictions. For example, the hospital may resent CDC's monopoly, "why CDC can confirm the diagnosis, but I can't?" Well, you know, the power of confirmation implies one's resource, authority, and benefits. Take tuberculosis (TB) as an example, wherever overlapped, hospitals and TB dispensaries are to be against each other, bringing their work corrosive effects. Of course, as neither of them wants to keep all on the slide, sometimes they will join hand, too; but, to offer the olive branch means showing the white feather. You come for me; oh, you must be more urgent; so why don't I grasp such a chance to suck in more profits?

(2) Other more profound considerations

Some volunteer groups hold that CDC and they differ in aims and objectives:

An epidemic calls for national inspection. It must be more like tracking. That is, confirmed AIDS patients should be closely shadowed until his end. As soon as patients die, it should be reported on time and that database should be synchronized. That's it, tracking and shadowing. But what CDC is actually doing is controlling.

Here is an old trick by CDC. From the very beginning, when they find the job vacant, they will encourage you to take it on; at that time, they are itching to make you conversant with this; but if you bargain for reward, they will leave your job to another free labour, at whom you may reasonably feel irritated. By driving such a wedge between groups, CDC racks up its profits. For this, I am convinced that being concerted will enable groups to assert their rights and interests, yet, I know, in the grassroots level it is such a big ask.

(3) Hospitals' concerns

Funds in the hospital are well guaranteed thanks to its administrator. Nevertheless, it is still worrisome in the long run, as its doctors said:

After all, the hospital is a self-sustaining business, having tried its best to meet the demand for funding. What's more, this institution is continuously losing money, for it should not only support its doctors but bear the high medical cost. What spurs the hospital and us to work is simply our conscience and public spirit; but passions, as always, won't last long. That explains why our boss doesn't impose on us sensitive performance evaluations. Even so, after a long time, few doctors will keep on. Some nurses are already reluctant to come. By the way, we have spent half a year applying for grants to treat AIDS patients. Sadly, no results.

AIDS is tricky because its medicine has certain side effects. We have to take precautions against lawsuits.

(4) Patients' counter-views

They think:

There is a national regulation that hospital—comprehensive or designated—should not deny patients medical care. It is regulated by our nation, albeit hardly executed in the grassroots level. So many times we have tried to figure out which one is to be blamed: the doctor? the hospital? Or, as some hospitals explained, people dared not to seek treatment from the hospitals who had performed operations on AIDS patients—if that's true, the society is to be blamed. Even so, I think, who would know the surgery except the hospital roared that out in the streets?! Also, HIV is much more fragile than TB; the operation should be fine with proper protection. Nevertheless, so wrong is the implementation of present policy.

The CDC is responsible for managing and tracking patients, while the hospital has no relevant duties but treatment. Indeed, the hospital, even though supervised by CDC, still makes no performance assessment on this issue. There, what means most is medical malpractices, and the shortage of patients is not a thing to doctors. In contrast, the CDC makes assessment, and its stuff will incur penalties if the infected turnover rate exceeds the standard. Of course, the hospital is pleasant to accept more patients for the sake of higher incomes, yet without these, anyway, it doesn't matter. But for CDC, it does matter; they are responsible for each patient who has not been followed.

Namely, few obligations are conferred on the hospital, and the hospital lacks the way to assess its service. One more thing, as for treatment, the hospital should impart more humanity so as to ensure patients' medical compliance. To be specific, for patients who resist medicine, doctors should expound its benefits along with the harm without it, and well inform these patients to take medicine on time. But being busy, doctors usually forget doing so. Worse still, since it is easy for us, the patients, to distinguish bad doctors from good ones, these kind-doctors, who may be on duty only two times a week, should accept forty to fifty patients each time, their clinic usually packed out, while those just-so-so-doctors, who may be on duty four to five times a week, should accept only four to seven patients.

All of the above should be perceived by the health department and then be solved. Their cause may not simply be imputed to the medical level or technology, instead, to a basic aspect. The hospital should systematize the protection for us.

(5) CDC's difficulties

Though CDC has offered great support to the volunteer group, yet nothing can they do for the treatment that patients care most. Also, since CDC is just responsible for those infected who haven't taken medicine, patients are in effect divided into two categories. These problems not only hinder the CDC itself and the volunteer group, but also bring harm to their cooperation. As CDC members said:

Funding is strictly regulated here, unable to be spent out of range. We can hardly support the volunteer group to do extra works, even though we know it is of great importance. Though we've reported these to the superior for many times, few executable plans could come into being. It is because the financial regulation is too rigid to change.

(6) Shared willingness of the three to communicate

Having analyzed the qualitative research, we can see the thee's common ends of AIDS prevention and treatment. Nevertheless, in their actual operation, they differ in their objectives and roles. To a large extent, it is such differences that cause their disharmony.

The volunteer group think:

In my opinion, "three-in-one", or "two-in-one", "eight-in-one", is mere hypotheses. It is pointless to roll all parties into one, cause in the end, people will work respectively according to his own duty. What matters most is a mechanism, or platform, for them to cooperate with each other.

The hospital:

Objectively speaking, we three work for patients and all strive to serve them better. Communication is surely important.

CDC:

"Trinity" may be the state that we want most. But how can we effectively communicate? We have no idea.

(7) Success in Tianjin

Its volunteer groups said,

Frankly speaking, we are enjoying sound and profound cooperation with our CDC. That's because we have circumvented every unnecessary procedure. Take NGO fast tests as an example, in many places these results are deemed invalid; one has to repeat the preliminary screening, the blood drawing, for recheck. But here, once examining a sample positive, we will directly send it for further confirmation, hence freeing patients from another onerous circle. Besides, patients may be apprehensive if the preliminary screening shows positive; then if asked to come again, he may escape. Considering that, CDC decides to recognize our test so as to ease subsequent works. Indeed, each place should have its own mode. For many areas, patients have to be drawn blood twice; but here, we avoid redundancy.

Though this mode was designed for Tianjin, we are accepting patients from all over the country. Maybe the organizations' service, including CDC's, is uneven among else areas. I'm surprised that a patient from Fujian should come here by plane for the CD4 test and then fly back. Another one, my acquaintance, should take four months in total to get his diagnosis; he precisely picked the bad days when CDC were on vacation, under decoration or on off-site meeting. As I joked, patients was reversely tracking CDC—but so many patients are tracking CDC; if I were them, definitely I would flee away with all my might.

Well, honestly speaking, we are just grouping our way. When cooperating with CDC in District A, we imitated our mode in District B. Luckily, it proved all right. We two have established an office in a public bath, providing people with immediate inspection service. Such cooperation, I hope, can be prompted in a larger scale, including CDC of other counties. Because for patients who live in remote area, traveling to the city is inconvenient; they may feel better if we can cooperate as well as we do in District B. Since we all intend to make it easier for patients, it is woefully sad to see someone waste his time flying here just for a test.

In my opinion, our institution demands diversified development, concerning that different groups are of their own feature. For example, my group commits itself to integrate patients with normal people; some may favor us, but some may prefer the group of pure patients. It depends on their actual demands. A copied mode from us may not be welcomed by those who wants the organization specializing in the positive.

Also, for NGO and CDC, I believe mutual trust is the most important. But presently, the two have formed a jungle, full of intrigue. For example, one organization of Tianjin, specialized in intervention, when cooperating with CDC on a project, was given the line that, they (CDC) could confirm the diagnosis but only in one certain day of the week and the sample must be sent before 8 a.m., or it would become overdue then be rejected. Things like that. (Q: Do you know why would they do that?) No, to be honest, we don't know. Facts are facts. Maybe, I guess, CDC members, recruited by public institution, responsible for over two hundred patients, are paid their salaries a certain amount; while we, in charge of just two patients, are paid the same.

(Q: Have you ever considered to make further cooperation with the urban CDC?) I lay it on the line—we have a tough experience with them. Why did I say from the very beginning that the ideology of a certain person would decide the attitudes of a section? In Tianjin, there used to be a CDC leader who bridled at our NGO, regarding us as anti-society and anti-government; then, perhaps due to some issues, he was dismissed. After that, good leaders, including the current one, came into power; now, we have few obstacles; we can even launch scientific projects.

I think the so-called "three-in-one" can be interpreted as an in-depth multilateral cooperation. Namely, instead of exploiting us (NGO) to collect blood samples, the CDC should apply itself to perfecting the connection between us. For example, we can succeed CDC on HIV screening or blood samples for recheck and confirmation, while leaving them still in charge of the last step; also, CDC can permit us to take over the epidemiological surveys and rechecks. In many places, CDC takes advantages of the NGO. But here, CDC rather assists us, and we have enjoyed such cooperation—may be bilateral—for quiet a long time.

But our connection with the hospital is not prolonged, also not smooth from the very beginning. However, the situation is able to be turned around if someone in certain position can takes his action with a firm attitude. So, strained though our relationship was at first, we and other organizations in Tianjin have successfully brought a wind of change. By now, we can say, we are working with the hospital.

However, to tell you the truth, our cooperation with the hospital can't reach the depth we have with CDC. The best we can do for hospital is to keep a long term connection with doctors, bring patients there and other odds and ends—far from the depth we have with CDC.

(8) A promising future

Before we came to Tianjin, pathetic voices were spreading among the society: the three sides are totally disjointed, as the CDC thinks highly of its bosses' opinion, the hospital wants profits, and the community group concerns its service objects; moreover, as the CDC is just responsible for managing, the hospital just for treating, and the group for improving patient's lives.

However, we got no such responses during our interview. On the contrary, this CDC doctor's opinion is more representative.

Actually, we three have common ground: the hospital finds patients; then the CDC cares and treats them; while the group can establish trust within their coterie, enabling its members to communicate better. You see, we two may hesitate during this talk, but they won't, cause they feel laid-back in their coterie. So, how about persuading government to unite the three into a circle? Then, the group can help patients enjoy the warmth of family, improving their lives; the hospital can provide treatment for patients copping body diseases; and the CDC can establish a mechanism for long-term management, giving patients preventative measures and HIV home-tests. However, to achieve that, there must be a leader. The government is the best to take it up.

Some of our patients are unwilling to be known to the group or any third party, saying: "doctor, you have got my phone numbers, but I hope no one else would know it." For those patients, the only thing I can do is exchange my numbers. People's receptivity varies, in great need of your regard. As I always say, in this job you should be genial and trustworthy enough so as to assure patients of his information secrecy. Now, medicine no longer controlled by CDC, patients are able to privately ask us for it.

Being relied on, I think we have done a good job. Some patients, even transferred to other provinces, still off and on call us to share their lives. Like: "I've been home, with a new spouse"—then I would reply: "do remember the protection"—he may say: "I'd worn the condom"—then I would praise: "nice, you protect yourself as well as others". That's all we can do for them, and that's because they trust you, not seeing you as a governmental worker.

Normally, there are more conflicts between doctors and volunteers. For example, the volunteer often visits the doctor along with heaps of patients, which is so exhausting for those medical workes. Besides, the doctor and the volunteer may have divergence on medicine. Plus other trifles. In the eye of CDC, is there any conflicts among your aim, the group's, and the hospital's?

So, the government should be coordinated with the hospital. Why would patients divide doctors into two types and exhaust the good ones? In a nutshell, there aren't enough doctors. If there were more, those doctors could spare the workloads, and hence have the time to instruct patients. But presently, they have to squeeze their words into heaps of patients.

I agree with such coordination: the government had better cultivate more clinicians. Presently, as doctors are overwhelmed by the patients, what can they do? Through empathy, it is easy to identify with both of them.

By the way, somebody attributes these to objective conditions—I disagree. Once the Health Authority orders, the Health Administrative has to immediately take action, even it is to expand the wards for outpatient.

2.3.6 Policy Supports for "The Trinity"

(1) A new perspective of thinking: the institutions

We need the humanity of doctors, but not of administrative functional departments. If a government puts its kindness into action, it often ends in restraint, management and regulation. For example, if the Project department set us a target, we have no choice but to work by the numbers: like, how many phone numbers to collect, how many of them to be valid; that's the only way for us to prove our work. We are pinned by those targets, then how could we root the true cruxes out?

Let's get back to cooperation. On account of the large amount of NGO in Tianjin, we are actually working with a group instead of a single entity. Although we welcome their cooperation, presently the question is, we just want their labour. Especially in our early phase, they are simply for completing the projects. Alas, all for fund; we need the group because we won't get money without those projects. What could we do when this capital chain ruptures—think about this year, the China-Gates AIDS Project, the Global Fund, both gone. Without cash, how could we maintain our operation? Right? And the special fund from the government should be distributed to NGO.

We can hardly further our cooperation with our CDC, at best tilting some resources. It is understandable because this CDC is extremely impoverished. Now, talking about the "three-in-one", I hold that it should rather be of two systems than two units. But in China, the NGO still lacks a mature system. For example, our patients from varied districts could all locate their accounts here They came for our sound cooperation with this CDC. It is not good, for in this case we can't popularize the good mode. We hope other CDC could imitate us, especially of our system. Especially the system. I hope that the cooperation between NGO and CDC could be built on their common interests—like a business—rather than superficial interactions. Uh, such interests may cause conflicts, too. For example, the CDC, recruited by public institutions, tends to be sedate, requiring our initiative. But it will be very helpful if they can offer us the olive branch. To sum up, we'd better extend our scope and bring a sweeping reform to the systems of NGO and CDC; if not, it won't be of wide significance.

The hospital prefers to remain aloof (from "three-in-one"). But its doctors and nurses are more moderate; they are highly approve of our NGO, but find few common grounds within our systems. Unlike that, we have a positive connection with CDC, both on system and business: for example, we often help CDC seek patients for testing. But in hospital, for doctors, only their skills will be assessed—though the "outpatients" may also be on the list, it won't be vital. So I think, we should focus on the hospital, not doctors. Because these workers will gradually know the problems, but only the institution can explore its demand for NGO and hence make a change.

(2) The government purchase service for the community group

We are wondering when the government will put it into practice. Although they have approved of it, the time and measures are still in bewilderment. Meanwhile, we have no choice but to continue doing stacks of work—medical test, psychological counseling—impossible to have a break.

Even though called the government purchase service, such cooperation should adhere to the principle of equality. But the government may see itself as an "employer". We understand, so mostly we will actively run for them. We will offer the olive branch to other organizations, but some CDC leaders, with peculiar ideology, may make things difficult.

(3) The mechanism to implement the policy

Actually, we can make breakthroughs, like a top-down system for the hospital. Premier Li Keqiang has approved of our NGO, but it's high time his stance made the difference. For example, we can stipulate that infection diseases hospitals should all conduct peers' service with NGO, or this measure cannot be implemented,

Because only by doing so can the hospital and its members be aware of this regulation, and then, to accomplish its target, they will at least spare offices for us when we come. That will be convenient for us. But now, we lack such binding rules. Well, of course, if there were too many inclinations to us, people may feel it unbalanced, doubting, isn't it too much? So, this is still under discussion. However, personally, I think it will be fine to put forward a few policies as a trial. For example, we can set a mechanism of reward and punishment in the non-designated hospital, punishing the one who refuses AIDS patients. Besides, we should appoint a supervisor—let it be the Medical Administration, Health Authority, or CDC, whatever. Without the accountability system and departments, all is but a dead letter.

(4) Performance reviews of CDC

There should be performance reviews in the CDC system. In previous projects, the wage was measured by the workload, not the quality. That means, how much I have done is how much I will get paid. So, if a worker was lazily satisfied and not willing to toil, he could still get his normal salary. That made diligence worthless and indolence safe. I regard it severe. Although CDC has implemented the performance review, it touched little; mostly the reviews are separated from the performance.

(5) Shared information

First of all, our resources are shared. How do we make it? When conducting consultation or test, we can collect all the contact details of the community. Then, during the preliminary screening, we can get a thorough data that CDC doesn't have. If they want, we will then give, but often they needn't, and trustfully leave it to us. We help CDC seek the HIV-positive, do follow-up visits and epidemiological surveys; while CDC, in turn, provides us with all the information on the National Epidemic Network.

Above all I've mentioned is about sharing information, then I want to talk about the cooperation by right of each own advantage. Primarily, the CDC is professional in HIV testing, while the NGO is uniquely tied with the community. If they can complement each other, I believe, it will be very helpful. Indeed, I've heard about some CDC who in their early stages harness groups to collect patients' contact information and then throw them away—as a matter of fact, however, in its late phase CDC is deeply mingled with the group. CDC has no way to supplant the group in peers' education.

So, it is important for each side to recognize its own fortes and look for the blend of each one's merits. For instance, NGO can provide humanistic cares, while CDC, being professional, can focus on the technology, such as CD4 testing, viral load testing, and drugs.

Personal opinion, when sharing information, the grassroots CDC often conflicts with the hospital. We had better let the urban CDC take the role of sharing information.

We should note that the CDC is able to share its information. But this institution has its difficulties – like, will NGO leak the information?—that concerns their principle. But in another way, if they admit to share a bit, it will help both of us a lot.

(6) Fast testing

Actually, our fast-testing here can immediately get the result, which CDC will take as the one of preliminary screening. In the meantime, CDC will spare its blood samples for us to do fast testing as a substitute for preliminary screening. Patients can hence avoid another turn of blood drawing. If we test one positive, we will send that sample to urban CDC for further diagnosis.

Firstly, the urban CDC sends the regional CDC reports in their lines of duty; secondly, we assist the regional CDC, together informing the results to the infected (as a matter fact, results precede reports); lastly, we, together with CDC, inform patients of the results.

(7) Not volunteer groups' monodrama

I think the crux of "three-in-one", in essence, is not all about the NGO. Instead, it is about the convergence and interaction among the CDC, the hospital and the NGO; whether they cooperate or not, we should see them as a tripartite unity of the same nature. Nevertheless, though the government is the most obvious and convenient one on this issue, people lay more stress on the NGO. Oh, it is what it is; you can't bend the one with more clout to your request—like us and the urban CDC. We must first be remarkable enough so as to attract their cooperation.

Talking about the institutions of three sides, I think each of them has its own feature. If we fused them together and take NGO as its prominence, a true mechanism would come into being, greatly deepening the three's cooperation. But presently, in Tianjin, the three haven't been interlocked as a complete circle, either solely between CDC and NGO, or between NGO and the hospital.

The CDC is level with the hospital. They have few intersections except some transfer between the leadership. Here we can see NGO's prominent function as a bridge. But we do expect that the CDC and the hospital can positively conduct more cooperation underlain by their own interests.

(8) Ways to strengthen the present cooperation

As a matter of fact, there are areas left for CDC and NGO to deepen their cooperation. For example, in Tianjin, the NGO often go to the infectious diseases hospital, but void of settled workplaces, they are just hanging there; while in Beijing, the hospital will prepare dedicated offices for NGO to make their work easier.

Commonly, people, though not infected, will be somehow timorous or reluctant to visit the doctor if alone in the hospital—and will concern a lot before leveling with doctors. So at this moment, I think the NGO is very helpful both for doctors and patients; NGO is the bridge.

I think patients can benefit from NGO in various ways. On the one hand, they will be more relieved to meet their peers before the doctor; on the other hand, they must be happy to have peers' company in every step. Because, you know, in China doctors was too matter-of-fact for patients. Although now their attitudes have improved a lot in infectious diseases hospitals, yet doctors, being superior, still make patients feel distanced, which may cause the infected serious mental burdens. They may fear HIV itself or discrimination, and may fall into depression.

(9) Necessity for strengthening the cooperation between CDC and hospital

We directly cooperate with the regional CDC. However, the urban CDC and the hospital, two administrations at the same level, have no right to manage each other. Thus, the document should only be issued by a higher health authority, like the health bureau; what's more, to ensure its effects, it should be with a fixed system of incentives and penalties followed by a course of actions. Now, we hope that the urban CDC could consider this, and then reach an agreement with the hospital or the health bureau, hence establishing a system for better work. We hope that someday there will be a mechanism, through which our voices could be heard by the regional CDC, urban CDC, and then the hospital.

By Harmonious Society, I think the fewer conflicts the better. Between the hospital and CDC, we'd better focus on the cause of these contractions. And in a sense, the hospital, due to its duty, has little power to do anything except treatment.

I'm puzzled that the hospital doesn't admit reports from CDC, not only on AIDS, but on other diseases like syphilis. Once in Tianjin, a patient, before taking medicine, was asked to do syphilis detection again to get the physical exam, but he had already been tested fine by CDC. As he related, the hospital didn't approve that result; they only recognized reports of other hospitals, excluding those of CDC. Some common reports, like on syphilis, are hardly recognized. There might be a few exceptions, but most patients have to resign themselves to experience all again. By the way, in fact, HIV and syphilis are tested according to the same tube of blood, but the bigoted hospital only admits the result on HIV. I guess, it is because the government has regulated that only CDC has such a right. But for that, the hospital would contribute another bother.

To be frank, such cooperation between hospital and CDC is really shallow. Well, of course, in recent years, things have improved a lot. We have established a sound relationship with the hospital, especially with its members like head nurses and attending physicians. Yet, the system we wanna build is in need of more efforts from the hospital and other sides.

(10) The lead of government; the communication to be the first step

We can apply various measures in parallel, such as mild advocacy, top-down managements, bottom-up responses, and radical stirs. Sadly, being NGO, we are always ignored no matter what we do. A simple example can be drawn. In the past, to get surgeon, patients were cornered to falsify their records, but it hadn't come to light until hyped up. For many issues, it is hard, really hard for the higher to deign to please us. Luckily, for all these years, we have managed to change something. We are longing for more winds of change to come as quickly as possible, because it is deciding the lifespan of patients. You should know, for the infected, time is life.

Meetings are always cordial where every issue is fine and dandy; whereas in reality, we are shunned—by the Social Security, for example. We also lack a lead. And the lead ought to and must be taken by a government sector instead of a functional one, because the later dares not excess the former, always under its pressure. Besides, regionally, the health authority should make a gesture first, specifying its policy and measures, or its attached departments won't take action. Moreover, that policy should be complete, or its loophole will shelter the negativity—just like the status quo. So, it is necessary to appoint one authority to enforce the whole process.

2.3.7 Criticisms to Broaden the Way

These interviews show that all the individuals can make suggestions at a micro level, but they cannot perceive themselves in a macro approach to these problems.

(1) Advice for the hospital: a normalized management

The hospital should see AIDS as a common chronic disease instead of a special one and hence provides normalized management. Then, the current practice on treatment costs should be abandoned, thereby putting all diseases into the insurance without exception. Because, on the one hand, only normalized management can maintain equality and respect; on the other hand, a "specialized" disease will bring patients only superficial benefits along with numerous discrimination, and will hinder the coordination within the hospital. We have submitted these proposals to the superior and the national experts, yet no feedback.

(2) Advice for the volunteer group: an individual-centered service

Some volunteers figured that the essential interaction between CDC and hospitals were rather patients than duty. Indeed, one should adhere to his principles or responsibility, but what we should ponder over now is how to provide more advantages for each patient. Take the social insurance as an example: presently patients may as well run amok for their rights; I am wondering why those related departments do not handle affairs together for those newcomers, which will help them conversant with the whole process. Unfortunately, now patients, without the volunteer group, have to plunge into sector after sector.

(3) Supplement: advice from the researcher

Firstly, the three sides can conduct direct communication in private, decide the lead, and then apply to the health office for a three-sides-forum for further negotiations. But they shouldn't ask the office for its direct participation.

Secondly, as for the theme of the forum, the three sides should speak out freely about their troubles in interests and their wants, exposing all the issues above board.

Thirdly, the forum is not to instantly solve every problem but to achieve mutual understanding on each one's circumstances and wants.

Fourthly, after the forum, the three sides should keep in touch so as to enhance their mutual understanding as well as the possibility to settle matters in cooperation.

Lastly, the three sides should bring forth a report which should then be sent not only to the health office but also to workers of each side. Thus, the three sides can jointly tackle the problems that even the health office is unable to solve in a short term.

(4) Reflections on the theory

In essence, all the trifles that we have met during the research are microcosmic problems of social management. They originate from the overall structure of our society that remains everywhere and have been the shackles on our community at large. Although macro-sociology can help us to better understand this, it is difficult to come up with concrete measures for improvement.

In accordance with the middle-range theory, the social exchange theory is the most applicable. To be specific, a new era is approaching as governments at all levels are positively conducting the "government's purchase service", but first we must equally treat the three sides as service providers and create for them an open, just and fair bidding system to compete. Thus, they will not end like "too many cooks in the kitchen", or "the Greek city-states before the Macedonia", but a trinity that supports the skyscraper of AIDS prevention.

2.4 Computerized Quesstionnaires, Interview Outline with the Three Sides, and Summary of the Qualitative Interview

2.4.1 Computerized Questionnaires

[Before starting, print and send the following to each respondent, asking them to keep it for themselves].

We are students and professors from the Sex Sociology Institute at Renmin University of China, and conduct this survey entrusted by Star of Haihe Working Group for HIV-infected People, a Tianjin volunteer group. We do not know you, nor your name and contact information; all your answers are so well-secured that even the volunteer group are unable to acquire them. You can fill out the following questionnaires at ease.

Withal, as a third part, we are independent from any institutions in Tianjin, having no bearing on any individual's interest. We are the only one to make analysis of all the data; and we won't handle them over to others.

The survey is charged by Professor PAN Suiming and Associate Professor HUANG Yingying (female) from RUC. If you find problems during the survey, you can inform them; if there are any damages to your interests, you can complain to them. Their phone number is 01082508956.

K01. Excuse me, would you like to answer the following questions?

1. Yes, I would.
2. No, I wouldn't. [skip to E11]

K02. To better secure your information, we want to make sure that you are answering questions in private. Now, if there is no one else around you, shall we start?

1. Yes, I'm ready. [skip to A01]
2. No, I'm not ready for that. [skip to E11]

A. Basic information

A01. Your gender.

1. Male.
2. Female.
3. Others.

A02. How old are you?

[two-figure number, ranging from 15 to 80, out of which the question will be repeated; if the error occurs again, skip to E11].

A03. What is your educational background (counting the present one)?

1. Uneducated.
2. Primary school.
3. Junior high school.
4. Senior high school, vocational high school, technical school or technical secondary school.
5. College degree.
6. Bachelor degree or above.

A04. How long have you been in Tianjin (including the suburb)?

1. Less than one year
2. Less than three years
3. Three to ten years
4. Above ten years

A05. Where is your registered residence?

1. In Tianjin, urban areas
2. In Tianjin, rural areas
3. Outside Tianjin, urban areas
4. Outside Tianjin, rural areas

A06. Would you like to tell us your current marriage status?

1. Unmarried, still single
2. Unmarried, but now cohabiting (same-sex)
3. Unmarried, but now cohabiting (opposite-sex)
4. Married, accompanied with a spouse
5. Remarried, accompanied with a spouse

6. Divorced.
7. Widowed.

A07. Have you had any work this month? (any works with payment, however long it is).

1. I have a job now. (farming is counted)
2. I'm still at school and haven't got a job.
3. I had a job before, but now I don't.
4. I have been laid off/ retired/ early retired, and have no job now.
5. I don't have any job in my whole life.

A08. How much is your monthly income (whatever the form) in the past 12 months?

[six-figure] (please enter the numbers in succession, and enter 0 if you have no income).

A09. At present, how many children should you support?

1. None
2. One
3. More than one
4. My wife (or I) is pregnant.

A10. Need you support the elders?

1. No, I needn't.
2. Yes, one elder.
3. Yes, two elders.
4. Yes, more than two elders.

A11. Have you already been in antiviral treatment?

1. I haven't been confirmed yet.
2. Having been confirmed, yet I haven't taken any medicines.
3. I have taken medicine for less a year.
4. I have taken medicine for one to three years.
5. I have taken medicine for over three years.

[1, skip to E01; 2, skip to B00].

A12. Which medicines have you taken by now? (multiple choice).

1. Zidovudine (AZT)
2. Lamivudine (3TC)
3. Stavudine (D4T)
4. Zhaxitabine
5. Deoxyinosin (DDI)
6. Nevirapine (NVP)
7. Delavidine (DLV)
8. Tenofovir (TDF)

9. Efavirenz (EFV)
10. Lopinavir (Creche)
11. Indinavir (IDV)
12. None of the above. I take others.
13. I don't know.

A13. How much did you spend for the drugs in the first month?

[six-figure] (please enter the numbers in succession, check it carefully, then you can press Enter).

A14. In 2012, how much have you spent on HIV medicines? (excluding the costs for opportunistic infection and health care products).

[eight-figure] (please enter the numbers in succession and check it carefully; then you can press Enter).

A15. Except drugs, what else have cost you for AIDS treatment in 2012? (multiple choice).

1. Trips and accommodations.
2. Referral, or transfer to another hospital.
3. Repeated tests.
4. Times lost while queuing up.
5. Health care products.
6. Treatments for opportunistic infection.
7. Others.
8. None of above.

A16. Could you tell us the total sum of your expenses of AIDS treatment in 2012?

[nine-figure] (please enter the numbers in succession, check it carefully, then you can press Enter).

B. Assessment of CDC's Service

B00. Here, we hope you could share with us about your opinions on CDC (Centers for Disease Control). Still, all your information is secured. Please fill in this questionnaire at ease.

(You can press Enter to continue after reading).

B01. Could you tell us which year you were tested positive? (please enter a four-figure number, such as "1998", "2005").

[four-figure, if the number is beyond 2013 or below 1982, repeat this question].

B02. Did you take that test in Tianjin?

1. Yes, I did.
2. No, I took it elsewhere. [skip to B4]

B03. Could share with us the exact address?

1. In CDC.
2. Through VCT (HIV Voluntary Counseling & Testing) arranged by CDC and the community.
3. In a infectious disease hospital.
4. In a common public hospital.
5. During blood donation/ transfusion.
6. In a private hospital/ clinics, or by a private doctor.
7. By the AIDS test paper by myself.
8. I forgot.

B04. Did they verify your identity during the preliminary screening? For example: you were to show your identity card, address or telephone number.

1. Yes, they did.
2. No, they didn't.

B05. Did you give them your real identity at the preliminary screening?

1. Yes, I did.
2. No, I didn't.

B06. Did they inform you of the results face-to-face?

1. Yes, they did.
2. No, they didn't.

B07. How were you informed of the results of the preliminary screening?

1. Via my telephone.
2. Online (like MSN).
3. Via the fixed-line telephone of my home.
4. Through neighborhood committees or units.
5. Through volunteer groups.
6. They came to my home directly.
7. I asked for it by myself.
8. Other approaches.

B08. How do you think the way you were informed? Will it leak your information?

1. Completely impossible.
2. Not likely.
3. Possible.
4. Very possible.
5. My information has already been leaked.

B09. Could you tell us how long was it between the preliminary screening and the day you were informed?

1. A week.
2. Half a month.
3. A month.
4. Less than three months.
5. Over three months.

B10. After the confirmation, who provided you with counselling in the first place?

1. CDC workers. [skip to B12]
2. Medical workers.
3. Volunteer group members.
4. Volunteers from other parties.
5. I searched advice on my own (by newspaper or online).

B11. By now, has CDC provided you with psychological counseling?

1. No, they haven't. [skip to B14]
2. Yes, but they didn't do so until I asked for it.
3. Yes, and they told me first.
4. Yes, they have, but I rejected that.

B12. What do you think of CDC's attitude during the counselling?

1. Very good.
2. Good.
3. Just-so-so.
4. Bad.
5. Very bad.

B13. Is the counselling helpful for you?

1. Very helpful.
2. Helpful.
3. Somehow helpful.
4. It's useless.
5. Not at all. I got false information.

B14. Have you tested your viral load of B14 after being diagnosed with HIV?

1. Never. [if selected, skip to B16]
2. Once in a while.
3. For several times, but not regular.
4. Irregular. But I wish it to be regular; I just can't keep on.
5. Regular, but the interval exceeds one year.
6. Regular, and the interval is around one year.
7. Regular, and the interval is less than a half year.

B15. Generally, how long would it take you between the virus load testing and the day you get its results?

1. A week.
2. Half a month.
3. A month.
4. Two months.
5. Three months or above.

B16. Could you tell us the reason why you didn't take the virus load testing after being diagnosed with HIV?

1. It is useless; it can't cure me.
2. It is not important.
3. It is a must, but not necessary to be regular.
4. I will take the test only when I feel sick.
5. It is not necessary since I have already been taking medicines.
6. It costs money, and I can't find a place to test for free.
7. I can't find an appropriate time and place to take the test.
8. Bad attitudes of the testing agencies.
9. Other reasons.

C. Assessment of the Hospital

C001. Here, we would like to listen to your opinions on the hospital. Still, all you information is secured, so please feel ease to fill in the questionnaire.

(You can press Enter to continue after reading).

C01. Could you share with us the year when you were informed to take medicines? Please enter a four-figure numbers, such "1998" or "2005".

[two-figure number ranging from 1982 to 2014].

[If A11 = 2, omit this question and skip to C17].

C02. Who was the first one to inform you of that (taking medicines)?

1. CDC.
2. The hospital.
3. The volunteer group (or its members).
4. Patients.
5. My family.
6. I acquired it on my own (by newspaper or online).
7. Others.

[if > 2, skip to C09].

C03. Who provided you with counseling when you were firstly informed to take medicines?

1. None. [skip to C09]
2. CDC.
3. The hospital.

C04. Are you satisfied with that counselling?

1. Very satisfied.
2. Satisfied.
3. Just-so-so.
4. Not satisfied.
5. Very unsatisfied.

[if < 4, skip to C06].

C05. Could you tell us what caused your discontent? (multiple-choice).

1. Bad attitude.
2. Improper time and places.
3. They asked me about my privacy.
4. It's too quick.
5. Its information is scarce, inaccurate or unreliable.
6. False information.
7. It lacks follow-up services.
8. Other factors.
9. I don't know.

C06. Before your first time taking HIV medicines, have you got other diseases?

1. Yes, I have.
2. No, I haven't.
3. I don't know.

C07. Before prescribed the first time, were you asked to have a medical check-up?

1. Yes, I was.
2. No, I wasn't, but they had inquired about my physical conditions.
3. No, I wasn't; they prescribe directly.

C08. When they were prescribing, did they give you the report on your physical check-up?

1. Yes, they did.
2. No, they didn't.

C09. As far as you know, is your combination of HIV drugs alike with others?

1. Exactly alike with all the patients.
2. Alike with over 80% of other patients.
3. Alike with around 50% of other patients.

4. Alike with only a few.
5. Alike with few.
6. I don't know.

C10. How was your CD4 count after you took your present medicine combination?

1. It rose sharply.
2. It increased slightly.
3. No big changes.
4. It dropped slightly.
5. It dropped sharply.

C11. At present, how is the side effect of your medicine combination?

1. Very severe.
2. Severe.
3. Not severe, tolerable.
4. Small.
5. Very small.

C12. How long was it, from the time you were diagnosed to take medicine, to the moment you actually got the medicine?

1. A week.
2. Half a month.
3. A month.
4. Two months.
5. Three months or more.

C13. Can you get every medicine on time during 2012?

1. Very punctual; every time is on time.
2. Relatively punctual; just sometimes earlier or later.
3. Not punctual; once in a while, I can't get the medicine for a long time.
4. Very irregular; I can never tell the exact time.

C14. At present, when will you go to the hospital to get the medicine?

1. Some working day specified by the hospital.
2. Some working day according to my appointment.
3. At weekend.
4. Anytime I want.

C14a. As for your privacy, have you encountered the following situations? (multiple-choice).

1. A large number of patients got medicines at the same time.
2. The hospital called my name in public.
3. I encountered my acquaintance.
4. I couldn't take the prescription in private.

5. Other situations that endangered my privacy.
6. None of the above; my privacy are well-secured.

C15. At present, do you feel convenient about the time to take medicines?

1. Very convenient.
2. Convenient.
3. I don't care.
4. Inconvenient.
5. Very inconvenient.

C16. At present, do you feel convenient about the place to take medicines?

1. Very convenient.
2. Convenient.
3. It doesn't matter.
4. Inconvenient.
5. Very inconvenient.

C17. When going to designated hospitals for HIV treatment, which situations below do you worry about? (multiple-choice).

1. My identity is exposed.
2. I am denied the operation or treatment.
3. I am forced to take unnecessary and repeated tests.
4. The cost of treatment goes too high; over-treatment.
5. Low level of medical care.
6. Poor medical conditions.
7. Bad nursing service.
8. Other concerns.
9. Nothing to worry about.

C18. In general, whose attitude do you prefer, CDC or the hospital?

1. CDC.
2. The hospital.
3. Both of them are good.
4. Neither of them is good.
5. I don't know.

C002. Here, we want to know the difficulties you have ever faced when going to hospital for other diseases (except the treatment).

(You can press Enter to continue when finish reading).

C19. Have you gone to hospital because of diseases other than HIV?

1. Never. [skip to D00]
2. Seldom.
3. Not often.

4. Often.
5. Very often.

C20. What kind of hospital have you gone to in 2012? (multiple-choice).

1. General community hospitals.
2. Designated community hospitals.
3. General hospitals.
4. Hospitals with infectious disease departments.
5. 5 Hospitals that can treat HIV.
6. Infectious disease hospitals.

C21. What concerns you most in the hospital? (multiple-choice).

1. To be asked about my diseases by an acquaintance.
2. To be interrogated by the doctor about HIV.
3. To be tested for HIV.
4. To be leaked information.
5. Referral.
6. To be denied surgery or treatment.
7. To be overcharged.
8. Other concerns.
9. Nothing to worry about.

C22. Have you initially told the doctor that you are an AIDS patient?

1. No, I haven't.
2. Yes, I have. [skip to D00]

C23. What makes you reluctant to tell the truth? (multiple-choice).

1. I may be denied treatment.
2. I may be overcharged.
3. My HIV-status may be exposed.
4. I may suffer from bad attitudes from medical workers.
5. It is unnecessary because they won't get infected.
6. Because they have no right to ask about it.
7. Whatever, they will examine everyone.
8. Other reasons.
9. I don't want to answer this question.

C24. Have you ever been tested HIV positive while seeing other doctors?

1. Never. [skip to D00]
2. Yes, I have, but only once.
3. For many times.

C25. Did something bad happen after you were tested HIV positive?

1. Yes, bad things happened.
2. No, nothing happened.

3. No, instead, nice things happened.

[if > 1, skip to D00].

C26. Could you tell us more details about those bad things? (multiple-choice).

1. They refused to treat me.
2. They asked me to make a referral.
3. They made a definite diagnosis, but didn't provide me with treatment.
4. I should be hospitalized, but they denied.
5. I was overcharged.
6. Bad attitudes from medical workers.
7. I quit my treatment and fled.
8. I was exposed.
9. Other bad things.

D. Assessment for Volunteer Groups

D00. Here, please share with us your opinions on the services of volunteer groups (the volunteer organizations). Still, all your information is secured, so please feel ease to fill in the questionnaire.

(You can press Enter to continue after reading).

D01. Do you belong to the community group for infected people or the hard-core of volunteer group? (either of them).

1. No, and I seldom connect with the group.
2. No, but I often connect with them.
3. No, but I am an activist.
4. Yes, I am the hard-core of the volunteer group.
5. Yes, I belong to the community group for infected people.

D02. In 2012, how many times have you participated in the group activity for the infected? [three-figure].

D. Judgement for volunteer group (volunteer).

D00. We are talking about how is the volunteer group's service (volunteer organization). All your answers are secret for the people inquiring you, so you can take it easy to answer. (When you finish reading, please press the enter key, and go on.)

D01. Are you a worker or a backbone volunteer in the infected community? Any organizations count.

1. No, I hardly contact with community groups.
2. No, but I often contact with them.
3. No, but I am an activist.
4. Yes, I am a core volunteer in the groups.
5. Yes, I am a group worker.

D02. How many times did you participate in the infected group activities in 2012? [___].

Whoever hosted the activities or whatever scale it is, it accounts if you have ever attended. If you have never attended, please answer "0".

[>0, please answer D04 directly].

D03. Why didn't you attend volunteer group activity? (You can choose more than one answer).

1. I do not know this organization.
2. I do not trust this organization or any person in the group.
3. I think it is useless.
4. I am afraid that it is not confidential.
5. I have some specific difficulties.
6. The volunteer group did not fit me.
7. The time or place of activity is not suitable for me.
8. Other reasons.
9. I do not know.

D04. Did volunteer groups (volunteer organizations) help you get the knowledge of tests, treatment, etc. Are you satisfied with it?

1. They helped me, and I was very satisfied with it.
2. They helped me, and I was rather satisfied.
3. They helped me, and I was rather dissatisfied.
4. They helped me, but I was very dissatisfied.
5. They did not help me.

D05. Did the volunteer group help you with psychological counselling? Are you satisfied with it?

1. They helped me, and I was very satisfied with it.
2. They helped me, and I was rather satisfied.
3. They helped me, and I was rather dissatisfied.
4. They helped me, but I was very dissatisfied.
5. They did not help me.

D06. Did the volunteer group help you with any specific thing in your own life? (Such as seeing a doctor, adjusting interpersonal relationship, and solving financial problems) Are you satisfied with it?

1. They helped me, and I was very satisfied with it.
2. They helped me, and I was rather satisfied.
3. They helped me, and I was rather dissatisfied.
4. They helped me, but I was very dissatisfied.
5. They did not help me.

D07. In terms of treatment, if the knowledge or information provided by volunteer groups is not the same with that provided by CDC or hospital, who would you believe more?

1. Volunteer group.
2. Centre for Disease Control, CDC
3. Hospital and doctor
4. I believe all of them.
5. None of them.
6. I cannot tell whom I believe more.

[If you choose 1, 4, 5, 6, please answer D09 directly].

D08. In terms of treating HIV, why do you believe CDC or hospital more than the information provided by the volunteer group? (You can choose more than one answer).

1. The group members are not professional doctors.
2. The information given by the group is not enough and shallow.
3. The source of information is not reliable.
4. The information doesn't suit me.
5. I know more than they do.
6. I do not trust the group or any of them.
7. I do not need any further information.
8. Other reasons.
9. I do not know.

D09. All in all, what have you obtained from the volunteer group?

(You can choose more than one answer).

1. Get knowledge and information.
2. Enhance confidence and promote mental health.
3. Make friends to avoid feeling lonely.
4. Get some specific help in life.
5. Learn to claim my rights.
6. I have some other gains.
7. I do not have any gains.
8. I do not know exactly.
9. I do not want to answer this question.

D10. We are still talking about the gains. Among all the gains from the volunteer group, please choose one that you think is the most important.

1. Claim your own rights.
2. Get some specific help in life.
3. Get knowledge and information.
4. Enhance confidence and promote mental health.
5. Make friends to avoid feeling lonely.

6. I have some other gains.
7. I have all the gains, but I cannot tell which one is the most important.

D11. From where you stand, what are the greatest advantages of volunteer group compared with CDC and hospital? (You can choose more than one answer).

1. Better attitude.
2. Higher quality of service.
3. More convenient and more prompt.
4. More considerate to me.
5. Easy to keep in touch for a long time.
6. More secret.
7. Other advantages.
8. Unclear.

D12. We are still talking about the same question. Compared with CDC and hospital, please choose one of the greatest advantages of the volunteer group.

1. Better attitude.
2. Higher quality of service.
3. More convenient and more prompt.
4. More considerate to me.
5. Easy to keep in touch for a long time.
6. More secret.
7. They have all the advantage and difficult to choose.

D13. Nowadays, the volunteer group is working on promoting the Tianjin subsistence allowances policy of AIDS patients. To what extent can you participate in this activity?

1. I cannot attend.
2. I rarely attend.
3. I can join in some activities.
4. I can participate more.
5. I can fully participate.

[>2, please answer D15 directly].

D14. What is the main reason that you cannot attend this activity? (You can choose more than one answer).

1. This activity cannot succeed.
2. I do not need such a policy.
3. I think this policy is not important.
4. I will attend if I can get paid or subsidy.
5. I do not have time.
6. I'm in bad health.
7. I do not trust the organizers of the event.

8. I have other difficulties.
9. I do not want to answer this question.

D15. Besides, volunteer groups are also working to promote the Tianjin AIDS patients' routine testing fee reduction policy. To what extent can you participate in this activity?

1. I can hardly take part in it.
2. I can attend a little.
3. I can join in some activities.
4. I can participate more.
5. I can fully participate.

[If your choice > 2, please answer D17 directly].

D16. Why do not you take an active part in promoting the Tianjin AIDS patients' routine testing fee reduction policy? What is the main reason? (You can choose more than one answer).

1. I do not have time.
2. I'm in bad health.
3. I do not trust the organizers of the event.
4. This activity cannot succeed.
5. I do not need such a policy.
6. I think this policy is not important.
7. I will attend if I can get paid or subsidy.
8. I have other difficulties.
9. I do not want to answer this question.

D17. Meanwhile, the volunteer group is still promoting Tianjin treating fee reduction policy of AIDS patients opportunistic infections. To what extent can you participate in this activity?

1. I can hardly take part in it.
2. I can attend a few times.
3. I can join in some activities.
4. I can participate more.
5. I can fully participate.

[If your choice is more than 2, please answer E01 directly].

D18. What is the main reason that you do not take an active part in the activity of promoting Tianjin treating fee reduction policy of HIV or AIDS patients opportunistic infections? (You can choose more than one answer).

1. I think this policy is not important.
2. I will attend if I can get paid or subsidy.
3. This activity cannot succeed.
4. I do not need such a policy.
5. I do not trust organizers of the event.

6. I do not have time.
7. I'm in bad health.
8. I have other difficulties.
9. I do not want to answer this question.

E. Stigma and Discrimination

E00. Could you please answer the question below that you once were discriminated against? It is all right if you do not want to answer these questions. We are still very grateful for your active participation and sharing.

E01. Could you tell us your route of infection?

1. Yes [please answer E03 directly]
2. No

E02. Why do you think you can't share your own way of infection? (You can choose more than one answer).

1. I cannot tell it how to carry HIV.
2. It won't help me even if I answer the question.
3. Because it is about sex, so I do not want to answer it.
4. I am afraid of being discriminated.
5. I am afraid of exposing other people's identity.
6. You should not ask this personal question.
7. This question itself is discrimination.
8. None of the above reasons are true. It is another reason.
9. I don't want to answer this question.

[Please answer E05 directly whatever you answer].

E03. Do you know your route of infection?

1. Yes, I am clear.
2. I am not sure, but I can guess it.
3. I do not know. [Please answer E05 directly]

E04. Which is your route of infection? (If you are not sure, please choose the most likely route).

1. Nosocomial infections (injection, blood transfusions, operation).
2. Unsafe sex.
3. Infected by selling blood.
4. Sharing of needles.
5. Accidental contact infection
6. Other ways.
7. Not sure.
8. I don't want to answer this question.

E05. Do you think there are stigma or discrimination for infectors in the present China?

1. No.
2. A little.
3. Little, but not serious.
4. Very serious.
5. Totally discriminate.
6. Unclear.

E06. Did you encounter stigma or discrimination by yourself?

1. No.
2. A few times.
3. Many times.
4. Very often.
5. Totally discrimination.
6. Unclear.

[If you choose 1 or 6, please answer E09 directly].

E07. Where did the discrimination you encounter come from? (You can choose more than one answer).

1. Government agency.
2. Medical institution.
3. Workplace.
4. Neighbour, native.
5. Family, relations, and friends.
6. Public opinion.
7. Inside the infected people.
8. Other aspects.
9. Unclear.

E08. The same with the last problem, please choose where did the most serious discrimination you had encountered come from?

1. Government agency.
2. Medical institution.
3. Workplace.
4. Neighbour, native.
5. Family, relations, and friends.
6. Public opinion.
7. Inside the infected people.
8. Other aspects.
9. Unclear.

[Female only, male go to E11].

E09. We come from the Institute of the Renmin University of China, specialized in researching sex. Therefore, we would like to talk about sex with you, and we will give you some payment for thanks. Could you please talk with us?

1. I do not want to talk. [please answer E11 directly]
2. I need to think about it.
3. Yes, I can.

[Female only].

E10. Thank you for your kindness, which is the greatest trust in us. Please look at the note which we sent to you before the survey. It contains the telephone number of Associate Professor, Huang Yingying (female): 010–8250-2956. She can come to Tianjin to talk with you. The time and place of the conversation are determined by you, and we will give you a payment.

E11. Thank you very much for your participation, and this is finished.

If you have anything else to talk about or complain the damage to you, please contact Prof. Pan Suiming and Associate Professor Wong Ying-ying directly (female): 010–8250-2956. If everything is ok, please return the computer to the investigator.

2.4.2 Outline of the "Tripartite" Interview

Research Topic: Problems and Countermeasures in "Trinity" Service Model of CDC, Hospital and Community Group in Tianjin.

Explanation: in the treatment of infected people, which role does CDC, hospitals, community groups play; how to promote better cooperation between these three parties.

Description required:

A. We only talk about work. There is no personal privacy involved.
B. We are just helping Haihe Star to complete the research. We are an independent third party, academic research unit, and students. There are no stakes with any side.
C. There will be no real name of any unit or individual in our final report.
D. I am totally amateur. Don't laugh at me, I study this subject for the first time. Please give me your advice.

What was your department responsibility for the work of people infected with HIV in the past?

If you have a sketch map of the division of labour, the provisions of the scope of work, and the responsibilities of each department or staff, could I take a picture?

What are your main responsibilities?

What are the main achievements of your own work?

What are the main achievements of your unit?

What aspects of your unit's and your own work coincide with the work of the CDC / Hospital / Community Group?

What specific work, in fact, should belong to your unit, or you can manage better?

On the contrary, which job should be done by (CDC/Hospital/Community Group replaceable)?

Which jobs are the most difficult for your own work experience?

Can you give a specific example?

To overcome these difficulties, for the arrangement of work in your unit, what else needs to be improved?

In your own or your unit's work, what difficulties and obstacles come from because CDC/Hospital/Community Group (replaceable) does not cooperate?

Can you give a specific example?

What difficulties or obstacles do you think cannot be solved by your unit? Who should handle it? How to handle it?

Probably there are comments or even complaints about the work of your unit/CDC/hospital/community group) What do you know?

What do you think of these comments?

What do you think your unit should do about these opinions?

what efforts have you or your unit made to coordinate these three aspects of work?

What else do you think should be done?

Do you think these three parties should communicate with each other in which way?

Overall service model of "Trinity" is just an assumption, what are your own questions, criticisms, suggestions and assumptions about it?

In a broader sense, what is your own opinion on the whole work of treating infected people?

In the period of dealing with infected people, apart from the good aspects, what do you think are their most unacceptable things or behaviors?

How should such a question be solved step by step? No matter whether we can make it. What is your opinion?

2.4.3 Frame of Qualitative Interview

A. Discrimination and being discriminated against

1. Institutional level; 2. Prevention more than treatment; 3. Unclear penalty provisions or lighter punishment; 4. The guarantee for medical personnel; 5. The management of hospital or medical service; 6. Actually being discriminated against; 7. Fear of being discriminated against; 8. Focus only on professional work, ignoring care; 9. Social misunderstanding and discrimination;

B. Privacy exposure and protection

1. It have been exposed; 2. Afraid of being afraid; 3. The possibility of being exposed; 4. The suggestions to protest privacy; 5. The behavior that not respect privacy; 6. The behavior of protecting privacy; 7. Not concerned.

C. Medicine taking

1. The production and reservation of medicines; 2. The distribution of treating expenses; 3. Research funding allocation; 4. Drug experience; 5. Get medicine; 6. Drug allocation

D. Detection

1. Over-examination; 2. Inform the results; 3. Detection of HIV viral load; 4. Detection of CD4; 5. Test before taking medicine; 6. Test before performing operation; 7. Detection of important health indicators; 8. Repeat detection; 9. Diagnosis; 10. Retention of documents; 11. Collection of testing fees; 12. Real-name testing report system.

E. Consultation and Prescription

1. Consulting before taking medicine; 2. Opportunistic infections counselling; 3.the quality of consultation; 4. Symptomatic treatment; 5. Change the prescription; 6. Comfort and psychological support 7. Prescribe the wrong drugs; 8. Prescribe expensive drugs; 9. Not familiar with the business.

F. Therapeutic conditions

1. Medical resources; 2. Medical settings 3. Health-care level; 4. Medical restriction; 5. Informed consent in medical treatment; 6. Service attitude.

G. Treatment process

1. Shirk one's responsibility; 2. Disguised shifting; 3. Refused directly; 4. Over-treatment; 5. Professional ethics.

H. The existence of volunteer group

1. The organization of fund sources; 2. Payment for volunteers; 3. Volunteer management; 4. The group needs financial support; 5. The group needs material support; 6. Mobility of infected persons from out of town.The status quo and suggestions of the "Trinity".

I. National policy

1. Policy publicity; 2. Compensation mechanism; 3 Competition mechanism; 4. Financial support; 5 Evaluation system; 6. Openness and transparency of policies; 7. Resource allocation; 8. Legal protection; 9. Management and implement of various policies and regulations.

J. For the aspect of infected

1. Trust expertise; 2. Trust medical staff; 3. Active cooperation; 4. Strengthen feedback.

K. In terms of community groups

1. Propaganda for target group; 2. Anti-discrimination campaign targeting the general public; 3. Community groups give suggestions more forwardly; 4. Providing information about the "comrade" group.

L. In terms of medical work

1. Overlap of work; 2. Staffing; 3. Support to volunteer groups; 4. Flexibility of work.

M. Tripartite coordination

1. Contradictions between the parties; 2. Coordination by superiors; 3. Coordination and cooperation in all aspects; 4. Whether the leader is present; 5. Communication and understanding; 6. The enthusiasm of all personnel.

Chapter 3
Sexual Transmission of AIDS

It is impossible to establish AIDS sociology without discussing the sexual transmission of AIDS. In particular, the author himself was able to participate in the study of AIDS precisely because of the study of "sociology of sex", so I have unshrinkable responsibility for studying sexual transmission. But this chapter is not pure theoretical speculation, but a summary of the experience of social. This can be divided into two parts.

(1) Quantitative analysis of the questionnaire survey results

It is based on the four randomly sampled "'All Sex surveys in China" of the total national population that the author personally hosted and implemented in 2000, 2006, 2010, and 2015 respectively. In order to make it easier for readers to read, the author introduces the basic information of these four surveys clearly at the beginning. Hereafter this text, it will be uniformly abbreviated as "Four National Surveys".

① Subjects and random sampling

The subjects of the four surveys are the total population in China between the ages of 18 and 61 who can read Chinese characters. In 2015, the total population of the country was 1.36782 billion, of which about 940 million were between 18 and 61 years old.

For details, see Pan Suiming and (US) William Bai, Wang Aili, (U.S.) Lauman: "Contemporary Chinese Sexual Behavior and Sexual Relations", Social Sciences Literature Press, 2004; Pan Suiming, Yang Rui: "Decade of Sexual Sex: A Tracking Survey of National College Students' Sexual Behavior".

Social Science Literature Publishing House, 2004; Pan Suiming, etc.: "The Empirical Study of the Success of Chinese Sexual Revolution: A Brief Report on the Results of a Random Sample Survey of the Adult Population in China: A Comparative Study of 2000 and 2006", Wanyou Publishing House, 2008; Pan Suiming, Huang Yingying:

"Sexual Change: The Sexual Life of Chinese People in the 21st Century", Renmin University of China Press, 2013; Pan Suiming: "2000–2015 Chinese Sexuality", (Hong Kong) 1908 Co., Ltd., 2017.

S. Pan, *The Social Construction of AIDS Issues*, A Sociological View of AIDS,
https://doi.org/10.1007/978-981-16-7519-5_3

The same data sources below this book are no longer indicated one by one.

National Bureau of Statistics: China Statistical Yearbook 2016, China Statistics Press, 2016.

Pan Suiming and Huang Yingying: "Sociology of Sex", Renmin University Press, 2011.

Random sampling survey is to ensure that among these 900 million people, no matter what kind of person, everyone is under equal probability of surveying. Not that there are many people of this kind and few people of that kind. Therefore, under ideal circumstances, a random sampling survey has 95% certainty, which is enough to represent the overall situation of these 900 million people.

Random sampling survey is the bottom line of all social surveys. If it cannot be done, there is no difference between surveying 100 people and surveying 1 million people. Each of them cannot represent the general situation of the Chinese people, and there will be very serious deviations.

Any kind of online survey cannot achieve random sampling. Therefore, no matter how many people are surveyed, it is very partial and it will seriously distort real life. We have specifically done a comparison between online surveys and field surveys, which is enough to prove this view.

Pan Suiming, Zhang Na, Huang Yingying: An Empirical Comparative Study of Website and Field: The Degree of Sample Deviation and Its Methodological Significance, Jianghuai Forum, Issue 4, 2009.

Based on national statistical data, such as stratified indicators of urban-rural differences, population scale, and divorce rate, multi-level equal probability sampling is performed. The primary sampling unit (PSU) is a county-level geographic area. Drawing the fourth-ranked streets and towns out firstly. Secondly, drew the fourth-ranked neighborhood committees or administrative villages, and finally equidistant sampling according to the total list of residents. Then extract the floating population according to the geographical sampling method. The result of the four national random sampling surveys is shown in Table 3.1.

② Method

Due to the high sensitivity of sex surveys, the author adopted the field survey method as follows. Investigators come directly to neighborhood committees and administrative villages across the country to conduct s for more than 3 days.

Do not conduct "household sampling", and do not conduct interviews at home, but directly sample individuals and invite the interviewees to the interview room prepared in advance, usually the room of the neighborhood committee or the school classroom.

Interview in a closed space: Make sure that there are only two people in each interview room: the investigator and the respondent.

The interview are between same-sex and one-on-one: Investigators are prohibited from interviewing the opposite sex.

Table 3.1 Brief introduction of the four national random sampling surveys (Excluding data from Hong Kong, Macau and Taiwan)

Project	Year			
Survey subject	People who can read Chinese characters			
Age group of objects	20–64-year-old	18–61-year-old		
Sampling method	Multi-level equal probability sampling			
Stratification criteria for sampling	Urban or rural area, population size, total industrial output value	Urban or rural area, population size, divorce rate		
Primary sampling unit, PSU/unit	60	120	103	103
Involved provinces, municipalities directly under the central government and autonomous regions	22	24	25	25
Sampling of survey site	Sample neighborhood committee or village with PPS method			
The number of terminal survey site	60	195	159	103
Urban neighborhood committee	50	150	123	67
Rural administration village	10	45	36	36

(continued)

Table 3.1 (continued)

Project	Year			
Sampling person from survey site	Sample residents and the floating population according to the geographical sampling method			
Total sample object	5000	6788	9992	7725
Attendance	3962	5688	7786	5601
Valid questionnaires	3812	5404	7202	5136
Proportion of male[a]	1899(49.8%)	2721(50.4%)	3433 (47.7%)	2472 (48.1%)
On-site effective response rate	96.2%	95.0%	92.5%	91.7%
Sampling effective response rate	76.4%	71.5%	72.1%	66.5%
Weighed factors of complex sample in statistic[b]	Urban or rural, gender, age	Urban or rural, gender, age	Urban or rural, gender, age, marital status	Urban or rural, gender, age, education

[a]In field surveys, the respondents are often less male and more female. Therefore, the higher the proportion of men in the surveyed subjects, the higher the quality of the survey.

[b]Complicated samples are the factors that first include stratified sampling in statistics: differences between urban and rural areas and different survey sites, and then include general demographic characteristics. This is the bottom line of statistics random sampling survey results.

The investigator and the interviewee had never met: the team leader came to mobilize, pre-invite and did not conduct interviews; the investigators could not know the situation of the interviewees.

Obtain the "informed consent" of the interviewees: Before the start of the interview, the interviewee should be clearly informed that the author would ask questions about sexual life, and he or she can refuse to answer any questions or quit halfway.

Interview on the computer questionnaire: Make the questionnaire into a computer program, and the investigator brings a laptop to the local area. After taught by the interviewers, the respondents complete the questionnaire alone by pressing the keyboard. This is currently the closest internationally recognized method.

For the details of the operation methods of the above four national surveys, the author wrote a detailed description of more than 20,000 words in Contemporary Chinese Sexual Behavior and Sexual Relations published by the Social Science Academic Press in 2004. The same methods have been strictly followed in subsequent s that conducted in 2006 and 2010 Readers can refer to the book, so I do not repeat it here.

③ Content

We investigate the interviewee about their social status, health status, charm and sex appeal, social interaction, love and sex of unmarried people, marital status (including cohabitation) of unmarried people, emotions of both parties, details of sexual life, non-marital relationship, multiple partners sexual behavior, "watch pornography", Internet activities, heterosexual massage, "one-night stand", sex life with street girls, exchange sex partners, multi-person sexual behavior, same-sex, multi-person sexual behavior, same-sex sexual behavior, sexual disorder, use of new drugs, purchase of sex products, sexual assault or sexual harassment.

If the respondent does not have certain circumstances, the computer will automatically skip to other question. Therefore, if the respondent does not have any sexual behaviors, then he will answer 86 questions; if he has all the circumstances, then he should answer 280 questions. In 2015, due to funding constraints, the survey content was reduced to at least 68 questions and a maximum of 192 questions.

④ Statistics method

All statistical analyses in this chapter processed by PASW Statistics 18.0 software. In the logistic regression analysis, dummy variables and control variables are set.

Part Two: Qualitative of Field Research

In this part, the author mainly presents the methods of "community" and "get-together" used by the author, and presents participatory observations and in-depth interviews of "red light districts", underground illegal "sex industries", and "street girls" and "male guesting". However, this book is not a monograph on this ground. The author only selected the research results on the sexual transmission. If readers are interested in further details, please refer to the author's relevant monographs (Suiming 1999, 2000, 2005; Suiming et al. 2005a, b; Suiming and Yingying 2008; Yingying and Suiming, 2008).

In this part, the author will not only present all aspects of the possibility of sexual transmission of AIDS in the underground "sex industry" in real life, but also explore how to treat these phenomena and situations from a sociological perspective and how to treat them better publicity, education and behavioral intervention for AIDS prevention. My purpose is to find some practical work method to create AIDS sociology.

3.1 The Risk of Sexual Transmission: The "Matthew Effect" of Men

3.1.1 Why Do We Study This Question?

As early as 1948, US Professor Alfred Kinsey insisted on including any kind of sexual activity enough for men to achieve orgasm, and to conduct an overall in his masterpiece. He said: "Regardless of whether you are studying an individual or a group, you must consider the multiple release channels of the subject, especially how much each of them contributes to the overall release status."

The research framework of "Sex Amount" proposed by Kinsey is undoubtedly a milestone in sexual research, but it is also an academic Pandora's Box, because it can easily induce future generations to come to the theory of "Ebb and flow". In other words, it is the increase or decrease of one or some sexual release pathways caused by the increase or decrease of other types of sexual release pathways.

In China, there are few specific terms and clear expressions for this opinion. However, it not only occupies a mainstream position, but also penetrates almost all related fields like mercury. It is even worse for men and various sexual activities.

For example, when we explain the reasons for the decline of men's sexual desire or reduction in sexual activity, it is believed that "someone will repay his debts at old when he owe it as young" means that there is too much sexual activity when you are young, and of course there is less when you are middle-aged. This is the "Understanding of ebb and flow" on the timeline.

The "ebb and flow" at the same period is more common. For example, when explaining the causes of adultery, Chinese people (and even many researchers) generally believe that it is mainly because some people are not satisfied with marital sex so that they will seek Extramarital affairs. Conversely, in the field of preventing the sexual transmission of AIDS, some people have been advocating "keep celibate". The premise of the reasoning is actually "more marital sex behaviors, less extramarital affairs".

In particular, the various comments on men's prostitution, whether it is the mass media or the research on AIDS prevention, implicitly assume that men have too few other types of multi-partner sex (usually expressed as "sexual depression"). Then they went to have sex with "street girls".

This is particularly manifested in the hypothesis of "pay attention to migrant workers and prevent AIDS": migrant workers are away from home and are unlikely to have other types of multi-partner sex in the city, so it is easier to go whoring. Similarly, for college students and teenagers, it is also because we assume that they are unlikely to have other types of sexual activities, such as extramarital affairs, so we are more worried that they will look for "street girls".

All in all, the false premise of "ebb and flow" of sexual activity not only easily affects China's AIDS prevention policies and specific work, but also has become almost common sense in Chinese life. This can only be broken through with rigorous empirical evidence. This is the main idea of this chapter.

There is little research on sexual relations (more than marriage or choosing a spouse) in our country's social sciences circle and the research on the sexual activities of men who are the main initiators and masters of sexual relations is even more limited.

Relatively speaking, the number of papers involving that men looking for "street girls" in the research on AIDS prevention in my country's public health community is on the rise. Nevertheless, owe to its professional limitations. these paper results still tend to treat it as a separate behavior.

However, the sexual transmission of AIDS through men not only comes from looking for "street girls", but also comes from other various types of male sexual relations and sexual activities, and the latter's transmission will become more and more serious. So, is there a connection between the two sides? What kind of connection is it? This is the question that the author studies.

3.1.2 *How to Make Hypotheses and Tests?*

This chapter assumes that there is a significant correlation between all kinds of multi-partner sexual activities of Chinese men and the number of sex transactions that tend to be "Matthew Effect". In social practice, this correlation is more likely: the increasing types of multi-partner sexual activities have significantly increased the number of sex transactions.

The test method in this chapter adopts multiple linear regression analysis. All models have been F-tested and collinearity results have been excluded. In order to save space, the statistical details have omitted.

The "previous year" referred in this chapter is 12 months before the survey, not the past year in the solar year. The "person times" mentioned in this chapter is based on the frequency concept of surveyed person: A with B is 3 times, and with C is 2 times, so A totally has 5 times.

In particular, the writer needs to point out that in the multiple linear regression analysis, the author takes the age of the respondent at that time, the length of education, the total monthly income, and the urban-rural difference of the survey location. These four variables are enough to reflect the most basic social stratification of Chinese men, which was introduced each model as a control variable. Therefore, all regression analysis results in this chapter are after excluding the effects of these four social stratification factors, that is, at the same level of social stratification, the "pure relationship" between the independent variable and the dependent variable. The design and use of control variables in our country's academic circles have not paid enough attention, so I pointed out it specifically. However, in order to save space, the analysis results of the control variables have been omitted.

(1) Sexual transactions

The male "sex trade" analysed in this chapter includes two activities. The descriptions in the questionnaire are as follows.

Find a "street girl": Now some "street girls" will provide you with sexual services if get your money, including not only sex, but also "hand job" (masturbation) and "blowing" (oral sex, blow job).

"Buy sex": Now some people give the other people some money or other benefits in exchange for sexual behaviors with the others, that is, "buy sex".

In common words in daily life, the first type of behavior is whoring, and the second type is "giving money" (including keep a mistress). The difference between the two sides does not lie in any qualitative difference in behavior, but in that the other person is a different person. Whoring is usually regarded as looking for a full-time "sex worker", while "buying sex" is the opposite.

The reason why I want to merge these two situations together is that from the perspective of the nature of sexual activity, these two are the same. Both are exchanged for sex life with money or practical benefits, and this is the only link connecting the two sides. This is enough to distinguish it from any other kind of multi-partner sexual activity, which a man might have.

The statutory documents of China's Ministry of Public Security are actually defined by this principle: "Unspecified acts of improper sexual relations between the opposite sexes or between the same sex, using money or property as the media, including oral sex, masturbation, and sodomy. Such acts are all prostitution and whoring".[1] In other words, "using money or property as a medium" is the nature of behavior, and the difference between prostitution and "purchasing sex" is only whether it occurs between "unspecified opposite sex or between same sexes".

The specific situation is shown in Fig. 3.1.

(2) Multi-partner sexual activity[2]

The definition of sexual activity is broader than that of sexual behavior, including those human activities that do not directly touch the body but still achieve sexual stimulation and satisfaction.

---

[1] In 2001, "The Ministry of Public Security's Reply on the Qualitative Treatment of Sexual Behavior Between Same Sex Mediated by Money".

[2] This concept was first used by the author in "The Role of Society on Individual Behavior-Taking the and Analysis of "Multi-partner Sexual Behavior" as an Example", "Chinese Social Sciences", Issue 4, 2002. Some people in the domestic AIDS research field also use the term "multi-sexual partners".

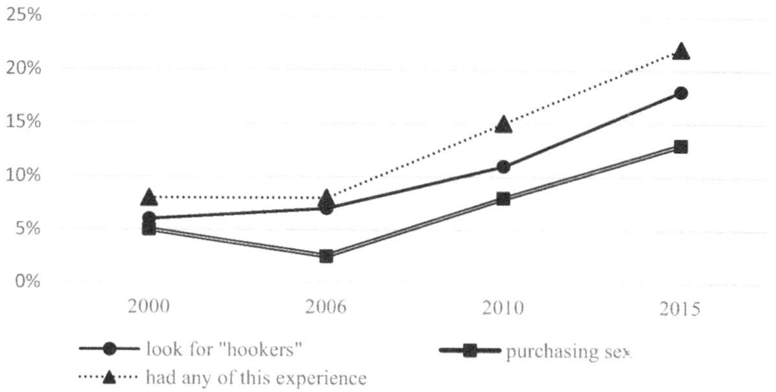

Fig. 3.1 The proportion of men looking for "street girls" and "buying sex" among men aged between 18 and 61

Multi-partner sexual activity refers to any kind of sexual activity other than a dedicated couple, no matter it happens simultaneously or sequentially, no matter who the other people is and what the result is, and no matter whether he/she is married or not.

This classification and concept came into being with the "AIDS era". It takes the number of sexual partners as the standard, and emphasizes that, regardless of marital status, as long as the object of sexual activity exceeds one person, it is a multi-partner sexual activity. This is because, from the perspective of the possibility of sexual transmission of AIDS, any kind of multi-partner and dedicated couple are essentially different. However, since the spread of AIDS among spouses in China has not yet shown up, this book has excluded the former couples of remarried, multiple married, divorced, and widowed people in the analysis of all multi-partner situations.

In traditional Chinese academic research and public opinion, there are only terms such as non-marital sex, extramarital sex, and premarital sex. They are all based on whether to get married (get a marriage certificate) as the criterion.

But from an academic point of view, marriage is just a social forced setting, and cohabitation of a spouse is the natural life entity of "marriage".

From the perspective of social reality, the current marital status in China is very complicated. Such sexual activities are increasing day by day: when they are unmarried but have sex, not married but cohabiting, between remarriage or multiple marriages, and after divorce or widowed.

According to the traditional definition, these people's current living entities have been judged to be non-marital sex relationships. If they have more partners, could it be called nonnon-marital activities? Therefore, the traditional definition is just the product of dogmatic values and a closed-eye thinking mode.

The specific situation is shown in Fig. 3.2.

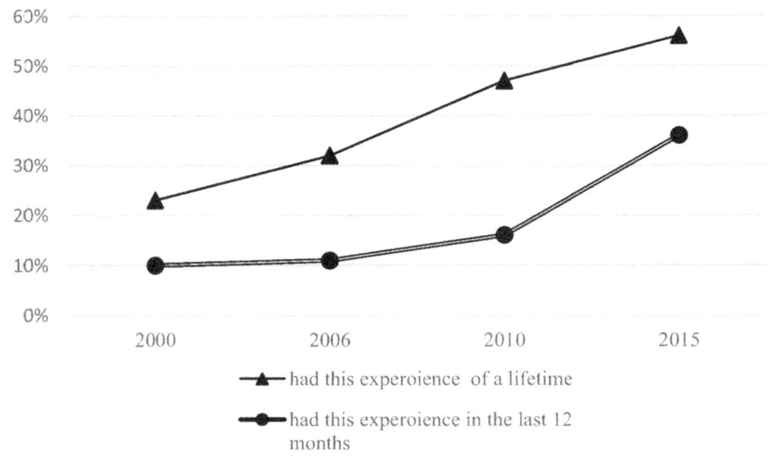

Fig. 3.2 Men's multiple sexual partner situation

3.1.3 Test Four Perspectives Separately, What Did They Find?

(1) Perspective 1: Comparison of historical development

Men's experience of multi-partner sexual activity is significantly correlated with the number of sex transactions in the past 12 months.

In this analysis, the definition of time is "in all one's life so far", that is, it includes the situation before the previous year. Some of these men have ceased certain sexual relations while others have not, and some men have only entered certain sexual relations since the previous year. Therefore, the significant correlation between these historical variables and the real-time variables of commercialized sex is enough to explain the author's above conclusion. In other words, men's multi-partner behavior not only tends to be a continuous development, but also tends to cross the confines like a rising tide.[3]

(2) Perspective 2: Comparison of sexual involvement

In the last year, there was a significant correlation between receiving "sex-related services" and commercialized sex.

"Sex-related services" mainly refer to the so-called "escort service" that involves paid dancing, watching pornography,[4] heterosexual massage for full body, and the

[3] Although the correlation is two-way interpretable, what is tested here is the historical existence and the situation of the previous year, so it must be a causal relationship.

[4] The author's definition in the questionnaire is: video tapes, VCDs (video discs), pictures, photos, books and magazines, pictorials, etc., which directly express the detailed content of sex life.

so-called escort service which includes accompanying guests to eat, drink and play.[5] Although Chinese law prohibits "paid escort services", it is also different from "prostitution and whoring". Correspondingly, "escort service" is exclude in the commercialized sex mentioned in this article. The degree of relying on the rapid development of the Internet. Sexual involvement is increasing, and sex transactions are undoubtedly the highest degree. This is the perspective of chain inspection.

The result of the multiple linear regression analysis is that the latter three have a significant causal relationship with the increase in the number of commercialized sex in the previous year[6]; coupled with the non-significantly related paid dance,[7] it just tests the existence of the chain development of the degree of sex-related activity.

(3) Perspective 3: Comparison of the degree of illegality

"Online sex activities" are significantly correlative with the number of commercial sexes in the previous year.

First, I have to explain "online sexual activity". In today's China, especially among young people, many sexual activities can expand to a remarkable social phenomenon only by "Online sexual activity" is sexual activities that can be achieved more widely and frequently through the Internet. Because there is no clear definition of it, the author had no choice but to create this phrase.

In today's China, sex transactions are illegal, and "online sex activities" are overlooked easily because of its "virtuality". Therefore, it is a good classification to examine the relationship between multi-partner sexual activities and sex transactions from the perspective of the degree of illegality.

The result of the multiple linear regression analysis is: Except for "nude chat on internet", all the "online sexual activities" investigated by the author have played a significant role in the increase of commercialized sex. On the other hand, if you can have more sex transactions that may be severely punished, then these "online sex activities" that are basically at the level of moral control will be a piece of cake.

This remarkable correlation is derived from a common feature of online sex activities and sex transactions: people have never known each other, and they form an instant sex activity through very brief and simple contacts. Therefore, the conditions and skills of interpersonal communication required to form these two kinds of sexual activities are similar, and it is easy to comprehend by analogy.

---

[5] In the questionnaire, the author defined "escort" as: not touching the genitals, more than having sex, just accompany the guests to sing, dance, eat, travel, swim, watch movies, etc., in order to make money.

[6] Here, the explanation of interaction does not conform to life experience, because most sex transactions occur during or after "sex-related services" rather than before, thus forming a causal relationship in practice.

[7] This is because nowadays dancing in China is mainly the "disco dancing" of young people without contact with each other instead of the old-style ballroom dance of physical contact. The relation to dance and age, the F test result (0.0000) can be corroborated.

(4) Perspective 4: Comparison of synchronic multiple types

In the past year before the survey, the multi-partner sexual activity experience played a significant role in increasing the number of sex traders. In other words, although some men had a lover, "kept woman", "a young seductress" or any kind of sexual partner of ordinary people in the last year, it did not prevent them from becoming more involved in the commercial sex.

Conversely, the increasing number of sex transactions will also significantly affect the occurrence of the other three multi-partner sexual activities.

(5) Summary

In the multiple linear regression of the above four perspectives, male various multi-partner sexual activities in different ages are significantly related to the number of sex transactions in the past year, and they tend to be a positive development trend.

If the quasi-causal explanation can be made unidirectionally, then the increase in the types of male sexual activity will play a significant positive role in the increasing number of their commercialized sex.

That is to say, under the same conditions of age, education, income, and urban-rural differences, if Chinese men's other types of multi-partner sexual activities increase, then the number of times they have engaged in sex transactions in the previous year will increase dramatically.

This is the Matthew effect and the result of its operating mechanism.

3.1.4 The Sociology of Sex's Explanation to Matthew Effect

First, concretely speaking, there is not only a close connection between men's multi-partner sexual activity and the sex trade, and it is not "Ebb and flow," but a Matthew effect.

Once men break through the system in any aspect, they would engage in more sex trading instead of just being satisfied with a certain type of multi-partner sexual activity. In other words, if multi-partner sex activities continue to flourish, even though China's current laws prohibiting prostitution have been unprecedently harsh, the growth of the sex trade will still go its own way, and the Matthew effect is likely to increase day by day.

The social construction mechanism of this Matthew effect is that China's current law to crack down on prostitution is just an extreme use of the marriage system to maintain a single spouse. However, the result of this two-pronged approach social setting is precisely that all things that it is trying to eliminate are all prosperous, but all things that it is trying to protect is damaged, and they all show the Matthew effect.

Second, from the perspective of countermeasures, the main route of sexual transmission of AIDS long been identified as prostitution. However, the current assumption that migrant workers, teenagers, and college students are high-risk groups is questionable. According to another analysis in this book, these people are far less likely to have multi-partner sexual activity than those who get rich first, the middle-aged married people, or urban upper-class men. In verse, if prohibiting prostitution has a long way to go, then the spread of AIDS in other types of multi-partner sexual activities by men will be serious, and it will first ravage the backbone of society.

Third, from an abstract point of view, biological factors only provide objective possibilities (essential conditions) for the composition of male sexual activity, while men's objective existence of whether has a spouse in society provides secular reality (sufficient conditions). But this is far from enough to explain the real situation, because the subjective choice of men and its results (the mutual increase of multi-partner sexual activity and commercialized sex) provide the possibility of development (Matthew effect), which constitutes the research about the third dimension-development conditions.

Fourth, the methodological significance of this cognitive result lies in: all social phenomena that we can investigate are not only objective existences that are inevitable under necessary conditions plus sufficient conditions, but also people's lives in their own life. People create variable value results actively. Without this perspective, any research is bound to take people and life as objective and static. Therefore, this book is the academic output of using "subjective construction perspective" (Suiming and Yingying 2007) advocated by the author.

3.2 The Risk of Sexual Transmission: Women's Multiple Sexual Partners

3.2.1 The Sex of Women in Social Networks

Since the 1990s, China's "sex revolution" has emerged, and changes in women's sexual relations have become the dominant aspect of this revolution. Because if China only has unilateral "sexual liberation" of men, then it can only promote the increase in "sex trades" ("street girls" who provide sexual service ordinary women have more multi-partner sex, and "selling sex" behaviors). Only if which may bring about more comprehensive changes.[8] Therefore, the study of women's multi-partner relationship has become an important aspect of understanding the current Chinese society and its development trend. It is a pity that the research on this subject in our country's academic circles is temporarily absent.

On the other hand, AIDS has been constructed as an important social issue in today's China. Sexual transmission has been identified as the main channel of spreading. If women have few multi-partner sexual relations, they are the terminal of sexual transmission and become the most innocent victims. However, if women's

---

[8] There is a saying in Chinese Ming and Qing novels that " men cheat like climbing a heavy mountain and women cheat like sticking a paper", which means that if a woman does not "take easy", it will be difficult for a man to succeed in cheating.

multi-partner sex increases, they will become a new starting point for sexual transmission. Finally, a wider epidemic of AIDS would be promoted.

Those men involved in the commercialized sex (the main source of spreading AIDS) act as bridge population for sexual transmission and bring AIDS to their female partners. As a result, the "virginity" of Chinese women has objectively become a barrier to prevent AIDS, and it becomes the key reason to explain the question of "why there are so few AIDS case in China". Whether it is the credit or sorrow of Chinese women, we should leave it for gender researchers to judge. What the author advocates is simply that the multi-partner phenomenon of Chinese women is worthy of further research, whether from the perspective of social network theory or from the perspective of AIDS prevention.

From 2000 to 2015, in just 15 years, the proportion of Chinese adult women who admitted having multiple partner sexual behaviors and the proportion of having had affairs both showed a huge increase, both of which have constituted significant difference in statistic (see Fig. 3.3).

Especially, in almost all social stratification included in the statistical analysis, the incidence of multi-partner sex and affair significantly increased. This shows that this change does not occur in some special group yet nearly all groups. This is also the main basis for the author's suggestion that Chinese women have also had a "sexual revolution".

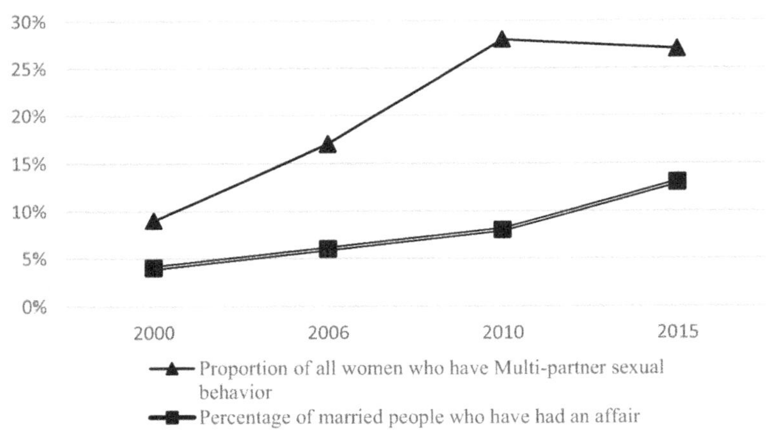

Fig. 3.3 The ratio of multi-partner sex and affair among women aged 18–61 in the country

3.2.2 *Hypothesis and Testing: What Factors Have a Greater Effect?*

As for the sensitive issue of women's multi-partner sex, people aren't just concerned about its historical development. They care about its reasons more.

(1) Hypothesis

In common public opinion, women's multi-partner sex is often considered as a personal moral choice. If there is nothing wrong with this saying in the traditional society, then, this situation has increased rapidly and has reached a considerable scale since the twenty-first century, so we must re-understand it from multiple perspectives.

As an exploratory research, this chapter assumes that women's multi-partner sex is the result of the joint action of social factors and personal choices. Therefore, this chapter mainly analyses which factors are significantly related to it.

(2) Inspection method

Logistic regression analysis was conducted with "whether there have been multi-partners for sex behaviour" as the binary dependent variable. All models have been tested by F-test and the results of collinearity are excluded. In order to save space, these statistical details are no longer listed.

From the results of regression analysis, it was clear that after controlling the differences between the two surveys, as a time interval, the self-reported incidence of multi partner sexual behavior of Chinese women in the twenty-first century has a significant correlation with many social factors, physical and mental factors and the subject construction of the parties. The most notable of these are the following aspects.

(1) From the Perspective of relative significance

First, other factors controlled, education level plays the most prominent role in women's self-reported incidence of multi-partner sex. Compared with women who have little schooling, the woman who get the higher level of education degree, the more possible to have multiple partner sex, and there are no exceptions. This can show that "female sex" is not born like this but is shaped like this; it can also show that although it is impossible to preach the correctness of multi-partner sex in any school in China, the more educated women are more indeed inclined to do so.

Second, the multi-partner sexes of married (in marriage), divorced and widowed women are extremely significantly higher than that of unmarried, cohabiting women. In another word, people usually have great hopes on marriage, which behave as a means of social coercion, and it does not actually fully play its role in blocking multi-partner sex.

Third, whether women are engaged in "sex-related entertainment" and "related activities" have played a prominent and extremely significant role. In other words, "doing or not doing something" has no less effect than "who you are". A woman completes her subject construction process by her own choices, or her subject construction results promote her to do something.

Fourth, the phenomenon of multiple partners tends to be done by urban wealthier women, because the two variables of "rank of residence" and "all monthly income" are extremely significantly correlated.

(2) From the perspective of the possibility of multi-partner sex

First, among all the factors included in the analysis, "generation" is the most prominent factor. Since the second generation, the possibility of multi-partner sex among women in each generation has increased significantly. This shows that under the same conditions, what kind of era and social and historical influence women are in when they enter puberty are inseparable from the possibility of their future multi-partner sex.

Second, the differences between women in different occupations are also very prominent. Compared with the very small number of women who do not know what occupation they are, almost all women with clear occupations are more likely to have multi-partner sex. Among them, female students and female workers in the business service industry are more prominent.

This may be mainly because such women have more conditions and opportunities for social interaction. In addition, the two types of women, female entrepreneurs and female leaders at all level, do not have significant correlation, maybe because they have more social problems. It is likely that the urban women who are under 25-year-old or unemployed lack the necessary economic conditions or social contact opportunities.

(3) Analysis of insignificant correlation

In many cases, the factors that are not significantly related in regression analysis tend to have more sociological significance.

Firstly, women's overall health status is not significantly related to multi-partner sex. Although several psychological conditions are significantly related, it is impossible to infer the possible causality, because we cannot know whether a woman is in a bad mood with multiple partners or vice versa. Therefore, the author can infer that the level of physical and mental health is not sufficient to explain why women have multi-partner sex.

Secondly, we can see that women think that "they are not very attractive to the opposite sex of the same age" and "do they really want to lose weight" (meaning "anxiety in figure"), none of them have any very significant effect on the incidence of multi-partner sex. Therefore, it is difficult to prove the hypothesis that "women who has messy private life are all vixens".

Once again, there is no significant correlation between whether he is a member of the Communist Party of China and whether he has too much multi-partner sex. This reveals the need to strengthen party discipline requirements for female party members.

3.2.3 *Multi-Factor Choices of Female Subjects*

The "sexual revolution" that has occurred among Chinese adult women since the twenty-first century can be explained by sociology. If many of the social, physical, and subjective factors listed by the author have undergone drastic changes and the status quo is indeed such, then it is obviously aimless to evaluate from the perspective of personal morality and may even add fuel to the fire.

Furthermore, if the changes and status quo of all the factors mentioned above are positive or unstoppable, then researchers and society will have to find new measurement scales and value judgement criteria.

3.3 Sexual Transmission Risk: Multiple Sex Behavior

3.3.1 *The Status Quo and Analysis of Exchanging Sexual Partners*

In today's China, it is often called "exchanging wives" or "exchanging spouses", but in this kind of sexual activity, the swappers are often not necessarily wives or spouses, but also chance encounters or sex workers. That's why I use the relatively rigorous term of "exchanging sexual partners" in this book.

In 2000, when the situation did not attract public attention, I did not begin investigating it. Since 2006, the questions in the questionnaire have been asked like this: Some people exchange spouses (or sexual partners) with each other to have sex. Have you ever done this?

A. Yes, I have.
B. No, I have not done this thing.
C. I can't understand this question.

The results of the survey are shown in Fig. 3.4.

Other factors play a more complex role so we need to analyze men and women separately.

(1) Analysis of men

According to the omitted logistic regression analysis, I found the following results.

First, there is no significant correlation between the possibility of exchanging sexual partners and any commercial sexual behavior This shows that swapping sex partners occurs more among ordinary people than in the so-called "sex industry", except the escort service. It is possible that the "escort" appeared and was accepted because that the two parties who exchange sex partners often meet or entertain themselves in recreational venues. The escort may even be one part of the people swapping sex partners.

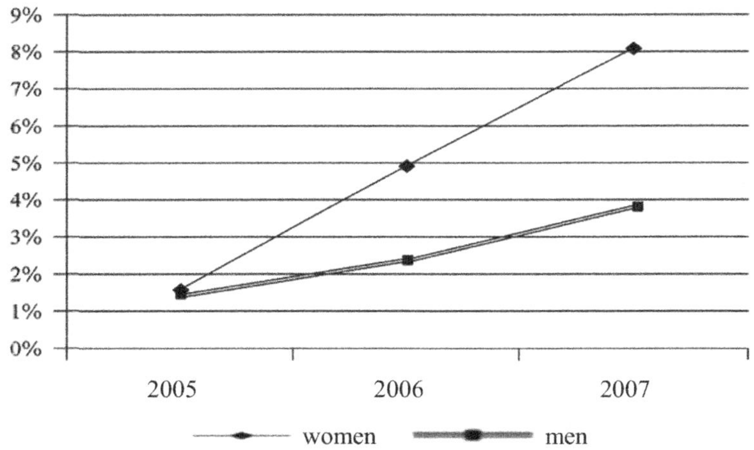

Fig. 3.4 Proportion of exchanging sexual partners

Second, the number of school years is the most significant social factor for men, but it shows a trend of inverse proportion. Only 0.6% of those with a college degree or higher education have ever exchanged sex partners, 1.0% of those who have attended high school, 2.2% of those who have attended junior high school, primary school and no school experience of the population is 3.3%. This is mainly because of the "sexual love control", that is, the more educated people, the more they believe in the existence of love and its restrictive effect on sexual behavior.

Third, the factor "marriage or cohabitation" has played a significant role, which shows that the sexual partners men exchanged are more likely to be their own spouses or cohabitants, rather than temporary sexual partners. Nevertheless, men who do not live in their own homes are more easily to exchange sexual partners. I can't yet give a satisfactory explanation for the paradox at this point.

(2) Analysis of women

The mechanism of women swapping sexual partners is quite different from that of men. According to the omitted logistic regression analysis, the factors that have had a marked impact are as follows.

Firstly, women who smoke 20 or more cigarettes a day are three times more likely to exchange partners. It may have nothing to do with physiological factors, as smoking more is likely to be one of the important manifestations of women's self-discipline and extensive communication.

Secondly, women who have had a "one-night stand" are 2.6 times likely to do so. It shows that breaking through "sexual love control" is the common feature of these two sexual activities, and it is especially effective for women. In this way, they have a significant correlation with each other.

Thirdly, women aged 30–39 exchange sexual partners most frequently, while those aged 18–29 and 40–49 rarely do so, and it was almost zero in 50–61 years old. As this should not be surprising, I won't go into the details.

Fourth, there are more social factors that have a notable effect on women than men: "socializing more than once a week", "not the highest-paid woman", and "not the floating population". These three factors greatly increase the possibility of women exchanging sexual partners. The explanation is that compared with men, this behavior of women is more subject to social constraints, rather than women's recklessness or boldness.

3.3.2 *Who is Doing Group Sex?*

In 2000, this phenomenon did not attract public attention. It wasn't until 2006, when it had been noticed, I started carrying out s.

The questions are as follows: There is a kind of sexual activity in today's society, that is, three people or more have sex together. Has that ever happened to you? (1. I have done this with a "street girl" or "sir" who serves sex; 2.I have done this with other types of opposite sex; 3.I have done this with people of the same sex; 4. I have never done this before.) The survey results are shown in Fig. 3.5.

Figure 3.5 shows that group sex is a small probability phenomenon in the total population of China, and it has not increased significantly in a decade. Because the proportion of women who have had group sex is too low to be in-depth analysis, the author will only analyze men below.

Among men who have this experience, about half have only done so with "street girls" who serve sex, and those that have done this with other types of opposite sex also accounted for half of the total. However, this simple percentage can't reveal a more in-depth situation. Then I conducted a regression analysis and found that in terms of social class, no other factors except for the "number of school years" of men played an obvious role.

From the perspective of personal characteristics, among the many related factors, only the variable "never go out overnight" can reduce the possibility of group sex. In other words, group sex is more likely to occur among men who go out for nights.

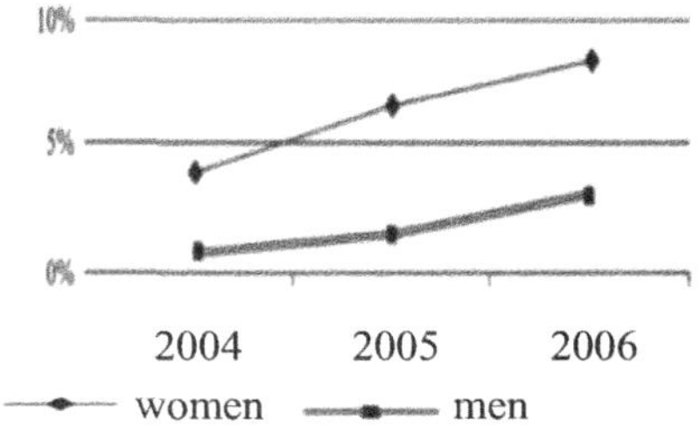

Fig. 3.5 Proportion of group sex

Commercialized sex has played a more prominent role. Whether men have "had sex with a professional street girl", "had paid for sex (to offer interests in return for sexual services)" or "had accepted the escort services", the possibility of men having group sex has significantly increased.

In addition, the factor of "having exchanged partners" greatly increases the likelihood of men having group sex, playing the most important role among numerous factors. This means that these two behaviors promote each other, and to a large extent, both of them have occurred. In other words, sexual intercourse among multiple people is a hurdle in the present Chinese society. Once someone gets over this hurdle, he may become profligate.

3.3.3 What is the Possibility of Sexual Transmission?

In classic or ordinary sexual behaviors, people praise one-on-one and condemn group sex. It is not simply a matter of sexual jealousy, but the deposition of monogamous history and culture.

Unfortunately, I can neither find the reason why they choose to exchange sexual partners or have group sex from the questionnaire, nor know the power relationship and interaction process between the two parties, let alone the results and subsequent effects. At the same time, it is also because the questionnaire survey itself is not suitable for analyzing any kind of small probability phenomenon.

However, if we denounce it as moral corruption just because group sex and exchanging partners are small probability phenomena, then no social science is needed. Otherwise, especially for the mass media, if its scale and social influence are exaggerated, then it also has nothing to do with social science.

What we need first is to recognize the reality, make factual judgments, and then discuss any practice or proposition. We need more reflection and should express our unique opinions firmly to promote the formation of a pluralistic society with the characteristic of "harmony in diversity".

As for the relationship between "multi-person sexual behavior" and the spread of AIDS, it can be so obvious, then I will confirm it by the results of random sampling surveys.

Among the total population of China from 18 to 61 years old, only 2.3% of those who had never "exchanged sex partners" taking the initiative to say that they had been infected with STDs. However, among those who have had such sexual behaviors, the incidence of STDs is as high as 20.2%, which is almost 10 times that of the former.

Similarly, only 2.2% of those who have never had "group sex" voluntarily told us that he once had STDs, but among those who have "had group sex with sex workers", it was as high as 34.1%, which is almost 17 times as much as the former. Among those who have "had group sex with other types of opposite sex", it is 17.5%; among those who have "had sex with people of the same sex", it is 25.0%.

3.4 New Risks of Sexual Transmission: New Type of Drugs

There have been some studies on the use of new type of drugs, but they are all partial and small-scale, and there are no representative studies on the general population. Based on the survey results of random sampling of the total population aged 18–49 in China in 2010, in this book, I attempt to analyze the overall situation of new drug use in China and the relationship with risky behaviors and self-reported sexually transmitted diseases (STI).

3.4.1 Current Situation of New Drugs

(1) How many people are using it?

According to data released by the Office of the National Narcotics Control Commission of China, there were 1,335,920 registered drug users nationwide by the end of 2009, of which 360,000 were abusing methamphetamine and ketamine synthetic drugs.

In our above survey results, those who reported that they had used new drugs accounted for 1.91% (136 people, standard deviation of 0.137) of the total population aged 18–61 after weighted statistics. The oldest person in the survey was 50 years old, so users accounted for 2.47% (136 people, standard deviation of 0.155) in the 18–50 years old age group.

By December 31, 2008, there were 528.89 million people aged 18–50 in China. Based on this calculation, the number of new drug users should reach 1.294 million. Considering the sampling error of 5%, the minimum number should be 1.229 million. This figure is 3.41 times that of government statistics. This is mainly because the number on the register mentioned by the government is actually the number of new drug users caught by the police.

Among the above-mentioned Chinese government's statistics: female drug users account for 15.4%. Our survey data is 16.9% (23 people, standard deviation of 0.000), slightly more than government data. This is also because it is more difficult for the police to catch female new drug users.

Among the above data released by the Chinese government, people under 35 accounted for 58.1%, but in our survey data, the average age of new drug users is 29.6 years old (standard deviation of 7.70; median 29), of which 18–34 years old accounted for 75.1%. This ratio is much higher than the data released by the government, because the police's ability to arrest is objectively limited.

(1) What kind of people are using it?

Since the oldest new drug user in our survey is 50 years old, this book will only analyze the situation of the 18–50 years old population.

We perform a chi-square test on the 8 most commonly used social stratification variables in sociological research and whether new drugs have been used. After obtaining the cross table (weighted Statistics), logistic regression analysis (dependent variable is binary variable) was conducted to find out which social factors played a major role. Since only 0.8% of women (N = 23, unweighted) have used new drugs, we only analyze the situation of men aged 18–50 (N = 3012, unweighted). The analysis results are shown in Table 3.2.

Through the analysis of Table 3.2, we find that among the eight variables, only marital status and monthly income are significantly related to new drug use. In other words, the main users of new drugs are unmarried and high-income men.

At the same time, since the above 8 variables are basically categorical variables, we also used decision tree analysis method (target category), and found the same result: Gain Percent of non-married men whose income is higher than the lowest 40% has reached 58%, plus married people, the Predicted Percent Correct can reach 100%. (Risk = 0.044; Std. Error = 0.004).

Table 3.2 Regression analysis of the relationship between the use of new drugs and social classes

Social layers	Sort	No drug/(%)	Sig	Odds ratios
Gender	Female	0.8		
	Male	4.2		
Marriage	First marriage and second marriage (in comparison)	1.7		
	Single	4.3	0.001*	2.465
	Cohabitation	9.0	0.000...	3.957
	Divorce and widowhood	2.1	0.000°	5.020
Monthly income	At the bottom 40% ((in comparison)	1.8		
	At the low-and-middle30%	2.3	0.021*	1.792
	At the medium-to-high20%	3.4	0.091	1.559
	At the highest10%	5.0	0.008**	2.217
Age	18–29 years old (in comparison)	4.1		
	30–39 years old	2.6	0.948	1.017
	40–50 years old	0.8	0.087	0.585
Profession	Out of job/at school (in comparison)	0.7		
	Take parts in all kinds of rural labor	1.9	0.901	0.927
	Workers, directly involved in production	2.6	0.883	1.078

(continued)

Table 3.2 (continued)

Social layers	Sort	No drug/(%)	Sig	Odds ratios
	Business and services	3.5	0.527	1.357
	White- collar worker	1.3	0.712	1.203
	Entrepreneur and leader	5.6	0.650	1.318
Degree of education	Primary school level and below (in comparison)	1.8		
	Junior high school level	3.1	0.745	1.139
	Senior high school level	2.3	0.872	1.068
	Colleague level	1.1	0.279	0.588
	Bachelor degree and above	2.3	0.651	0.788
Place of residence	Towns (in comparison)	2.4		
	County or county-level city	2.6	0.522	1.197
	Prefecture-level ciity	2.7	0.667	1.132
	Provincial capital	3.4	0.959	0.982
	Municipalities	1.3	0.155	0.339
Fluxion	Permanent residents (in comparison)	2.4		
	Migrant population	2.6	0.098	0.694
Constant value			0.000	0.018

3.4.2 New Drugs Endanger Overall Health

The analysis results of new drugs and health are shown in Table 3.3.

Table 3.3 shows that the use of new drugs is not only closely related to drinking and smoking, but also brings serious psychological problems to the users.

3.4.3 New Drugs Severely Increase Sexual Transmission

It includes: ① multi-partner behavior; ② condom use; ③ self-reported incidence of STIs. The analysis results are shown in Tables 3.4, 3.5 and 3.6.

From Table 3.4, we first find that compared with no-drug users, the users were more likely to have risky sexual behaviors, and it's true in all the sexual relationships we have observed. This is very shocking.

The table ranks new drug users' risky behaviors from high to low according to the result of F-test. Among them, the risky sexual behaviors (exchanging partners, multi-person intercourse, same-sex intercourse, and "buying sex") with the highest increase in new drug users are precisely the behaviors that have the greatest probability of spreading AIDS. In other words, the degree of new risks brought by using new drugs to the spread of AIDS is much greater than the various figures listed here.

Table 3.3 Cross-analysis of new drug use and health behavior

Cases	Options	No new drug use (%)	Have new drug use (%)	P-value	Sig.
Drinking	Never drink	99.5	93.9		
	Drink, but never drink too much	0,3	3.8		
	Rarely drink too much	0. 1	0.0		
	Usually drink too much	0. 1	2.3	58.519	0.000
Smoking	Never smoke	43.2	22.9		
	Smoke less than 10 cigarettes a day	25. 1	30.5		
	Smoke 10–19 cigarettes a day	19. 1	27.5		
	Smoke more than one box a day	12.6	19.1	22.306	0.000
Be afraid of getting old	Very	8.6	14.5		
	A little	26. 1	36.6		
	Not very much	28.0	26.0		
	Not	37.3	22.9	17.354	0.001
Being down in spirits	usually	6.9	16.0		
	sometimes	65.8	66.4		
	never	27.3	17.6	18.682	0.000
Feel tired without any cause	Usually	8.9	16.8		
	Sometimes	64. 6	64.9		
	Never	26.5	18.3	11.701	0.003
Get angry easily	Usually	6.6	13.7		
	Sometimes	58.4	57.3		
	Never	34.9	29.0	10.398	0.006

Table 3.5 shows that users of new drugs use condoms more only in long-term sexual relationships, and there is no obvious difference in non-marital relationships. But they obviously have more non-marital sex behaviors than others, so their current level of condom use cannot reduce the chance of getting AIDS at all.

This shows that the use of new drugs has greatly increased the possibility of the spread of STIs and AIDS.

However, the current prevention work in China is mainly focused on injecting drug users, which is far from enough. Although the users of new drugs may be more scattered and hidden, the sociology of AIDS, which is being established, is more

Table 3.4 Cross-analysis of the use of new drugs and various multi-partner sexual behaviors

Sexual relations	Specific circumstance	No new drug use	Have new drug use	F text	Sig.
Exchanging sexual partner	In last year	4.05%	28.2%	152.981	0.000
	Number	1.56	2.76	1.997	0.160
Group sex	In history	6.2%	33.1%	137.706	0.000
	In last year	4.2%	26.0%	127.679	0.000
	Number of occurrences in previous year	2.71	5.61	6.582	0.011
Gay sex	In history	2.1%	17.6%	114.500	0.000
Selling sex	In last year	4.1%	24.4%	112.321	0.000
	Number	1.64	7.15	7.861	0.006
Multiple partners (last year)	There has been	39.6%	71.0%	60.242	0.000
	Number	1.08	3.56	71.600	0.000
	Have new sexual partners	16.8%	45.8%	72.642	0.000
	Number	1.97	3.45	12.497	0.000
Multiple partners (last month)	There has been	12.9%	36.6%	60.409	0.000
	Number	0.23	0.84	45.487	0.000
	Have cross-sexual partners	39.6%	58.3%	7.768	0.000
	Have new sexual partners	7.6%	25.2%	51.299	0.000
	The number of new sexual partners	0.96	1.29	1.970	0.161
Multiple partners (in history)	There has been	58.5%	90.8%	55.509	0.000
	Number	3.30	14.52	65.678	0.000
Doing sex with "ladies"	In last year	10.9%	34.4%	67.021	0.000
	Number of occurrences In previous year	4.69	10.60	71.759	0.000
"Purchasing sex"	In last year	9.4%	30.5%	61.181	0.000
	Number of occurrences In previous year	3.30次	4.87次	2.165	0.142
"One-night stand"	In history	14.4%	34.4%	39.291	0.000
	In last year	8.9%	25.2%	38.284	0.000

(continued)

Table 3.4 (continued)

Sexual relations	Specific circumstance	No new drug use	Have new drug use	F text	Sig.
	Number of occurrences In previous year	1.36人	3.69人	14.392	0.000
Extramarital settings	There has been	32.9%	61.9%	23.140	0.000
Full body massage from opposite sex	In last year	22.6%	51.9%	60.272	0.000
"Jerk off"	There has been	11.6%	39.7%	91.130	0.000
	Number	2.18次	7.57次	30.826	0.000
Accept "escort"service Dancing consumption	In last year	19.0%	50.4%	77.917	0.000
	Number	1.39次	7.63次	64.971	0.000
	In last year	44.7%	73.3%	41.703	0.000
	More than ten times	6.4%	25.2%	74.641	0.000
Touching the vaginas of dancers	There has been	19.9%	40.6%	23.092	0.000

Table 3.5 Use of new drugs and condoms

		Always (%)	Usually (%)	Seldom (%)	Never (%)	P-value	Sig.
Do it with long-term sexual partners	No drug use	12.9	14.6	29.5	43.1		
	Drug use	36.2	19.0	2.07	24.1	29.234	0.000
Purchasing sex services	No drug use	67.4	10.1	15.0	7.5		
	Drug use	45.0	20.0	25.0	10.0	8.118	0.044
Do it with "ladies"	No drug use	66.8	18.4	9.2	5.6		
	Drug use	68.6	8.6	17.1	5.7	3.512	0.319
Buying sex services	No drug use	46.2	17.3	21.2	15.4		
	Drug use	59.1	13.6	18.2	9.1	1.166	0.761

Table 3.6 Self-reported STIs

Situation	Options	No drug use (%)	Drug use (%)	P-value	Sig.
Venereal disease	There have been	4.8	32.8	175.618	0.000
The time of getting venereal disease	Within the past 12 months	0.9	15.3	167.445	0.000

likely to make new contributions in this field by using its own unique and research methods.

3.5 Theoretical Discussion: Sociological Solutions on Sexual Transmission

The reason why sexual transmission becomes an "issue" rather than just a biological phenomenon is that it occurs among people. And it can be transmitted to different people in different social situations and activities. The person who has been infected are likely to be very different from the transmitter. In other words, AIDS is spread by people under certain social conditions, thus it has become a "problem" in the Sociology of Sexuality research. Let's analyze how the sexual transmission of AIDS exists in society.

3.5.1 Sexual Communication of AIDS is Networked

The concept and corresponding theory of social network of sexuality were first systematically discussed by Edward Lauman, John Gaggon and others in the Social Organization of Sexuality which was published in October 1994.

Figure 3.6 shows a schematic diagram of social network theory of sexuality. The basic meaning of this concept is that human sexual relations are not entirely one-to-one. Some people maintain sexual relations with more than one person at the same time. For example, A only maintains a sexual relationship with B, but B maintains

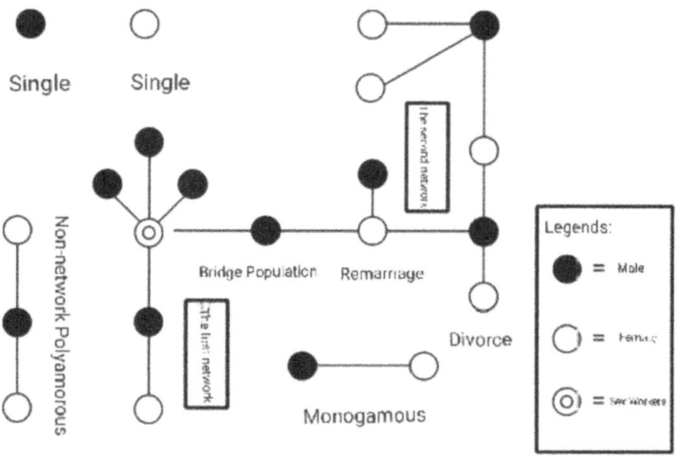

Fig. 3.6 Schematic diagram of social network theory of sexuality

a sexual relationship with C and D at the same time. In this way, A, C and D form a 4-person sexual social network through B. If any one of them still maintains a sexual relationship with others, then this sexual social network will expand even more.

In real life, such small social network of sex can often be seen. Moreover, if someone in network A has a sexual relationship with another one in network B, then these two networks are connected together. If many members of a community or group maintain sexual relations with more than one person, then many of this community or group will be connected to the same sexual social network.

Of course, there are many people who have no sexual partners at all, so they are a solitary point on the distribution map of the social network of a certain community or group, and they are not connected with anyone. Those who both only have sex with each other are shown as a single-line structure connected by two points and isolated from others on this map.

The social network theory of sexuality comes from the path theory and analysis method in sociology. It is so important because it puts forward an assumption that the same person will have different sexual behaviors when having sex with different people. For example, when a man has sex with his wife, he may be gentle; when he has sex with a lover, he may be passionate; and when he is a whoremaster, he may be rude. Moreover, for different people, the specific sexual intercourse methods he uses may also be completely different. The same is true for women.

Starting with this hypothesis, social network theory of sexuality believes that in previous studies of sexology, people's sexual behavior is often regarded as the actor's own affairs, ignoring the influence and effect of the other party on the actor. It is impossible to explore the actual situation when people have sex in real life. It also believes that when studying any sexual phenomenon of human beings, the research subject must be put into his (her) sexual social network. Only by exploring the different behaviors of the actors in different network locations can we fully and deeply discover the real situation of the actors' sexual behavior.

The sexual social network composed of different sexual relationships is just a manifestation of itself. In addition, there are social networks of sex in terms of sexual concepts and sexual morality. For example, A tells C and D that a certain sexual phenomenon is good after learning it from B. Then in terms of the learning of sexual concept and the spread of sexual morality, A, B, C, and D constitute a sexual Social network. Individuals exchange information with multiple people in such a certain sexual social network. He masters social norms by learning from one person, and adapts to the whole society by getting used to someone.

Undoubtedly, from the perspective of sexual sociology, the social network theory of sexuality is very cutting-edge. It not only emphasizes that an individual's behavior comes from the feedback of the other party and is restricted by the social environment, but also stresses the path through which social morality and sexual rules, etc., restrict and affect everyone Therefore, after it was put forward, the traditionally saying "sexual behavior" no longer only refers to individual's independent behavior, a kind of networked sexual behavior, which is in the interaction between individuals and society, and restricted by learning and feedback.

The social network theory of sexuality is also called "sexual theory in the age of AIDS." As the theory of sexual network in it is very conductive to studying the transmission path of HIV, to finding out various methods that may block this path, and to estimating the possible transmission range of AIDS. It is based on this theory and its analysis method that lawman and others radically pointed out that it is difficult to spread AIDS in large scale among heterosexual population, and the main energy and resources of AIDS prevention work should be placed on high-risk groups.

The proposing of social network theory of sexuality indicates that the sexual sociology has passed its initial stage and has begun to grow into maturity. It enables further development of the theory of social determination of human sexual behavior in sociology of sexuality, and provides the theory with a more realistic and specific basis. In terms of practical application, in addition to preventing AIDS, this theory also provides a reasonable, feasible and solid theoretical foundation for the social management of sex and the self-awareness of unique sex groups.

3.5.2 "Bridge Population" for the Spread of AIDS

This is first related to our understanding of "sexuality." In the past, AIDS prevention work often started with natural science and always regarded "sexuality" as individual behavior. But here is the reality:

First, sexuality is not individual, but happens between two people in most cases, and from the perspective of sociology of sexuality, it occurs in social networks. When you have sex with someone, how do you know if that person has had sex with someone else? Your partner's sexual relationship with another person will definitely affect your sexual relationship. Isn't that simple?

Second, sexuality is more than just a behavior. Public health workers always emphasize that the key to preventing AIDS is to change sexual behaviors. In fact, the biggest risk of not wearing condoms is not AIDS, but love! Most of the two people in love do not use condoms. You don't trust me? Or I don't trust you? The same goes for "street girls". A "street girl" will 100% use condoms when having sex with her whoremasters, but she will never use them with her boyfriend. Condoms mean mutual distrust and suspicion. This turns sexual relations into bargaining, into a frictional movement of cylinders. How can this happen to love?

When it comes to the spread of AIDS, from a sociological perspective, the prevention of AIDS must be mainly aimed at "Bridge Population", rather than simply aimed at "street girls". Usually we assume that "street girls" are the source of infection, but who spreads AIDS to those "just debut" girls? A study in Thailand found that the proportion of whoremasters with sexually transmitted diseases is much higher than that of "street girls." This is not from reasoning, but after based on collecting all the condoms used in the brothel and testing them one by one. So, who is the culprit?

Even if a certain "street girl" is a HIV carrier, and three whoremasters have had sex with her, then she has spread the virus to these three men. This is right. But if these three men have never had sex with other person, then only these four people will be infected in total, no more, and no further transmission through sexual channels. However, if one of them has a wife, the fifth person may be infected. This man will spread AIDS as a bridge between people. If this man has multiple-sex partners, he may spread AIDS to more people. This is how sexual social networks are connected. Among them, it is not the "street girls" who play the most important role, but the bridge population.

If AIDS were limited to drug users, homosexuals, and illegal "sex industry" participants, China would never have so many HIV-infected people. The number of people in the above groups is limited. Even if there is a 100% infection rate (in fact, it is no near that high), there will never be such a large number of AIDS patients, and it will not grow so rapidly. The accelerated spread of AIDS is entirely due to the "Bridge Population" connecting the participants of the illegal "sex industry" and the general public, who have nothing to do with each other.

Then who is the most important "Bridge Population"? Our survey results show that 26.7% of men in the so-called "early-prosperous class" such as factory directors, managers, and bosses have engaged in prostitution, and the proportion of whoremasters among them is 10 times that of urban male workers and 22 times that of rural male workers. In addition, they also have the highest number of other female "sexual partners", 1.95–2.60 times that of male workers and 2.87–3.37 times that of male farmers.

China's current AIDS prevention policy basically focuses on drug users, homosexuals, and illegal "sex industry" participants, but it has never been mentioned in a single word that it is necessary to provide condom education to factory directors, managers, bosses, etc. In fact, the easiest way is that before all companies and enterprises are registered, their legal persons and senior managers must receive AIDS prevention training first. Some public opinion is always propagating that it is sexual liberation that caused the AIDS epidemic. However, the real culprit is actually this kind of "Bridge Population". They not only engage in whoring, but also have multi-partner sex, having mistresses, acting as sugar daddy and even raping female workers. It is them who spread AIDS on a larger scale.

By extension, can we really "care about ourselves" in the spreading network of AIDS? In any kind of sexual relationship, should we still believe in the "loyalty hypothesis" (assuming that the other party has no other sexual partners)?

3.5.3 Sexual Transmission Depends on the Social Structure

(1) Sexual transmission under social policy

From the perspective of AIDS prevention, AIDS is most likely to be spread through group sex, followed by "sexual intercourse" (penis inserting into vagina). That is to say, the risk of other sexual activities is small and diminishing.

In this regard, why not focus China's limited police, material and energy resources on "sexual intercourse", the main goal of AIDS prevention?

(2) Sexual transmission in social management

As the large-scale "anti-vice" campaign continues, "street girls" will be fined if caught. As the "street girls" are poor, and it is impossible to ask their families for help, they can only borrow money from the "procuress" or their bosses. As a result, even in the free-employment sex service places, a "street girl" will become a debt slave. In order to repay the debt as soon as possible, she can only "do business" harder. How can she prevent AIDS in this situation? How can it be possible to say "I will not do it without a condom" to whoremasters?

In particular, there are no secrets in the illegal "sex industry". Those whoremasters who come frequently will soon know which street girl is a "debt slave" and will have more unscrupulous sex without condoms. It dramatically increases the risk of sexual transmission.

(3) Sexual transmission in customs

In some places, there is a superstition among some men that "having sex with a virgin is auspicious". They believe that it can bring them good luck. I have repeatedly heard of this situation in fieldwork, but have no chance to interview any of them. In the word of mouth, business men seem to be more likely to believe this statement. In this case, they will never think of AIDS prevention.

Among the participants in the illegal "sex industry", especially among the whoremasters, there is another saying that "Complement of Yin and Yang", that is, the secretions of both parties must achieve futunio and harmony in sexual intercourse before they can "benefit themselves". This will obviously reduce the use of condoms.

(4) Sexual transmission in folk beliefs

"Penetration worship" is very popular among Chinese men, which means that sexual intercourse must be penetrated, otherwise it is not "sex". Therefore, the reason why whoremasters do not use condoms is not simply "wearing a condom will affect sexual pleasure". The most important thing is how they define "sex" and "sexual intercourse".

The traditional cognitions of many whoremasters are: ① Wearing a condom is no longer a real sexual intercourse which means the male's penis firmly attached to the female's vagina without hindrance; ② Wearing a condom means "losing", which is equivalent to no sexual intercourse.

(5) Sexual transmission in hierarchical status

The fear of being "lowly" always shrouded "street girls'" heart. As a result, they will have two diametrically opposite perceptions about using condoms.

In the eyes of some "street girls", the reasons for not using condoms are that condoms are a sign of "street girls", will block direct contact with the body and cause gynecological inflammation; in addition, this will also offend old whoremasters because it is difficult for them to have erections after wearing them.

But some other "street girls" think that using a condom can show that they are just "doing business" rather than having real sexual intercourse; and this can also "block the dirty things of men".

Some "street girls" even think that wearing a condom is to show their identity as "street girls" which can prevent themselves and whoremasters from having feelings with each other. The basis of this view is that condoms are only used between "street girls" and their whoremasters; in any other sexual relationship, no one would use condoms.

(6) Sexual transmission in "self-taught" whoremasters

In the process of investigating low-class whoremasters, I learned about the strategies of whoremasters dealing with sexual transmission: look (look carefully beforehand), smell (check whether there is an odor by smelling it), touch (stretch his hands into the vagina and touch it), and wash (ask the street girls to clean their internal and external genitals in advance). Under the guidance of such knowledge, none of the whoremasters surveyed used condoms and they even ridiculed that wearing condoms was stupid.

(7) Sexual transmission in collective activities

In the of whoremasters, I found that wearing a condom is an interactive behavior in a circle. If a "leader" uses condoms in a specific small circle, other men in this circle will pay more attention to him. Reverse the process. Otherwise, the probability of using condoms will be greatly reduced.

(8) Sexual communication in intimate relationships

China's current AIDS prevention work is basically aimed at high-risk groups. However, in the age of "sexualization" in the twenty-first century, the multi-partner of ordinary people is increasing rapidly. Although it has been put on the agenda, the prospects of condom use between husband and wife are really bleak.

Between lovers or couples, no matter which party proposes to use a condom, it means that they have been unfaithful, or that they suspect the other party of "unfaithfulness". In this way, it is difficult to maintain the relationship between these two parties.

(9) Sexual transmission in diverse genders

In today's China, money boys are increasing day by day, so do the "cross-dressing" sex workers. They have a greater risk of HIV transmission than heterosexual intercourse.

(10) Sexual transmission in different interpersonal relationships

Our publicity and education work on AIDS prevention can no longer assume that people like a blank sheet of paper, know nothing about AIDS. In fact, the Chinese people have a clear recognition of the risk of AIDS. The risk of a certain sexual relationship is directly proportional to the use of condoms. This situation is fully demonstrated in Table 3.7.

The percentage of couples using condoms during sex is 7.1%; 10.7% with other sexual partners; 48.4% for "buying sex"; 49.0% for "selling sex"; 64.2% for prostituting. People who have used it last time accounted for 80.2% of total.

Table 3.7 Percentage of condoms used in different sexual relationships

Sexual activity	The proportion of always using condoms (%)
Conjugal sex life	7.1
With other sexual partners	10.7
"Purchasing sex"	48.4
"Sell sex"	49.0
Men have sex with "ladies"	64.2
Have used it last time	80.2

That is to say, our publicity and education should shift from condescending lessons and intimidation to discovering, summarizing and promoting the successful experience of ordinary people in condom use.

(11) Sexual transmission in differential pattern

Although they work as "street girls", they will adopt different sexual lifestyles in illegal sex transactions, in intimate relationships in love, and between couples. They will choose to wear condoms or not. Researches all over the world have found that although "street girls" may insist on using condoms in illegal sex transactions, they rarely use condoms in any kind of dating relationship or husband and wife relationship. Sexual relations with different natures indicate different relationships between people.

Similarly, men will adopt different sexual life strategies in different sex relationships, including whether to use condoms. This is not only reflected in the research results, but also a common sense in the male world.

3.5.4 *Risks Come More from the Illegal "Sex Industry"*

In the 13 "red-light districts" investigated by me and my team, there are four main forms of illegal "sex industry": "slavery", personal attachment system, free employment system, and self-management system.

Regarding "slavery", everyone may have seen the report of "a virgin jumping off the building" in newspapers or television. A girl who was deceived to a certain place and forced into prostitution jumped off the building and was seriously injured.

We had investigated on the spot and saw the whoremasters, who is a female boss. The real reason is that the underground "sex industry" practiced "slavery", forcing and detaining "street girls" who had no personal freedom at all, no wages, and no fixed commissions. They were rewarded instead. The organizers constituted actual prison in the form of anti-theft nets and anti-theft doors.

Another form of organization is the personal attachment system, which exists in most cities' hair salons and massage places. Its characteristic is that the "street girls" must live in the workplace which generally provides them meals, but this is different from slavery. Under slavery, "street girls" have no personal freedom at all. "street girls" in the personal attachment system are free during non-working hours, however, they can't live without this specific business place. Because if they stand on the street, the police will arrest them. This shows that the most important part of illegal "sex industry" is place. Without venues, sex transactions cannot happen.

This is also reflected in the "anti-vice" practice. We recently completed a research project to explore the evolution of the "anti-vice" policy since the 1980s. At the beginning, it was always aimed at "street girls", the same with today's AIDS prevention work, and then directing at the bosses and "pimps" of the underground "sex industry". In 1999, it started targeting places, which took Mafia-Like gangs as protective umbrella. Then rectifying and governing the "backstage" had became a key point. I think they will realize one day that this is actually a corruption problem. As long as the corruption problem exists, the problem of the underground "sex industry" cannot be solved.

Whoremasters are linked with "street girls" in these places, without which "sex industries" cannot function. Most of our AIDS prevention workers go to "street girls'" living places for publicity and education. This is extremely absurd in logic. Government will continue the "anti-vice" work. Although you promise that your is only for academic research purposes, will the bosses and the "street girls" believe you? As long as you stay in the venue, you may see the sex trade. In the past, the highest penalty for organizing, hosting, and forcing others into prostitution in China was the death penalty and a large number of bosses and "pimps" have been shot. You threaten their lives directly, how could they cooperate with you? However, if you talk to a "street girl" when she is shopping, it is impossible for her boss to interfere. Under the personal attachment system, the boss only cares for "street girls'" activities during working hours,, it has nothing to do with the bosses who they go shopping with or chat with.

The feature of the free employment system is that the "street girls" don't live in the business premises, which is similar to our daily commuting. It practices the "hunger discipline" and no one forces the "street girls" to be whoremasters, but they will be no income if they don't do that.

The characteristics of the self-management system are self-employment, voluntary employment and fully responsibility for its own profits and losses. Self-employment "street girls" often work as "chatting servicers", "female netizens" and "botty calls". In some areas, there have even been cases in which several "street girls" hire a "procuress" in partnership, and the power relationship between these two parties is completely reversed.

To put it vividly, "slavery" existed in B.C. 200 years ago about the personal attachment system, 20 years ago about the free employment system and 2 months ago about the system of self-employment. Why does every young man want to be a small boss whenever he has a chance, and not want to be a white-collar worker anymore? This is because they are personally free.

The biggest side effect of China's current "anti-vice" campaign is that it subconsciously encourages "slavery". The more powerful the "anti-vice" campaign is, the more scared the whoremasters are. As a result, the bosses have to use various methods to attract whoremasters. The first is advertising that there are all virgins, as a result, these young street girls are easily forced into prostitution. The second is that for safety and concealment, they have to work 24 h a day, which means the "street girls" cannot leave and lose personal freedom. In addition, after being caught and punished, the "street girls" can only turn to the bosses or "pimps" and "procuresses" for help. As a result, they are easier to fall into the abyss of "slavery" economically and personally. In particular, according to the "Prostitution Law", even forced prostitution is also an offense, so how many forced "street girls" dare to escape and ask the police for help? Our in Sichuan found that this is the most effective weapon for "slave owners" to scare young street girls. Don't these objectively encourage "slavery"?

Under this "slavery" organizational form, it is a fantasy for social scholars or medical workers to promote AIDS prevention to bosses and "street girls", for whom AIDS is really just an extremely minor matter.

Different organizational forms will inevitably lead to different personal behaviors of the members. Everyone knows that whoremasters don't like to use condoms, and they often use them only at the urging of the "street girls". However, the "street girls" who are trapped in "slavery" or personal attachment do not even have the minimal personal freedom, so how can they ask their whoremasters to use condoms?

Current surveys of epidemiology and preventive medicine always ask about the frequency of condom used by "street girls". Why not ask whoremasters the same question? This is a typical gender issue. Most of the participants in this type of survey are women who lack gender awareness. When you ask questions like this, you assume that the "street girls" are victimizers. If they do not use condoms, they will transmit AIDS to their whoremasters. Conversely, if you ask "street girls" about the frequency of condom used by the whoremaster, the premise immediately changes. That is, if a whoremaster doesn't use a condom, he will transmit AIDS to a "street girl". This is the awareness of gender equality.

Is there any equality between the "street girls" and the whoremasters? The whoremasters are rich and powerful and don't care about moral conscience at all. However, most of the "street girls" under "slavery" or personal attachment system leave their homes for city for the first time. They may have studied in elementary school for only three years and have no sense of law or equality. How can there be equality between them and the whoremasters? AIDS prevention workers have carried out many activities to educate "street girls" to use condoms, and they get it, but when whoremasters refuse to use condoms, they don't even have the right to say this! What is the effect of your promotion of AIDS prevention to "street girls"?

In the sex trade under "slavery", as "street girls" are originally persecuted and deceived to do that, whoremasters are more likely to commit violent rape. As a result, it is prone to bleeding during sex and the probability of getting AIDS increased greatly. All the whoremasters know that the "street girls" under "slavery" have no rights, so they have no scruples. Such prostitution is not a commercial behavior, but a complete rape.

Such "street girls" are even less likely to acquire knowledge and skills on AIDS prevention. They are all in a semi-closed state and have no personal freedom. Where can they obtain this knowledge? Let alone the rate of seeking doctors and treatment for STDs. How can they go to see a doctor when they are not free at all? After getting STDs, she has an increasing the probability of getting AIDS. Especially, they will ignore the value of life even more because they have long regarded their bodies as an accurate measurement of economic units. The prevention of AIDS is too far away from them.

Another important route of AIDS transmission is drug abuse. The "red light districts" where "slavery" is practiced are also high incidence areas of drug abuse. When these two behaviors overlap, the probability of AIDS infection becomes much greater. Bosses who practice "slavery" are usually sheltered by local Mafia-Like gangs and turn a blind eye to "street girls" taking drugs. However, the other three organizational forms of the illegal "sex industry" have some "rules" that can "help" us prevent AIDS.

First, "street girls" are never allowed to take drugs. "Procuress" and "street girls" are very strict with each other. Whoever of them takes drugs will be fired immediately. This is because whoremasters believe that drug-addicted "street girls" will deceive, steal, and even kill them for their money. The whoremasters are all local influential people. If they know that a "street girl" is taking drugs, they are sure to smash this shop. Unfortunately, few AIDS prevention workers have thought of using this point to carry out their work.

Second, once a "street girl" gets STDs even if the whoremasters don't know it and she can continue to work, she will be immediately looked down upon by other "street girls" and "procuresses". Otherwise, she may even be swept out because of her stupidity. For "street girls", sexually transmitted diseases are firstly a very embarrassing thing, which is related to their status in the group, and secondly this is a health issue. AIDS prevention workers can actually take advantage of this point.

Another point is that "street girls" are generally more afraid of AIDS than we think. If we publicize its harm to them once again, it will be so superfluous. What we need pay attention to is that many of their understanding of AIDS is wrong. For example, many "street girls" believe that kissing will spread AIDS 100%. So where does this fallacy come from? It is a summary of their professional experience. They have sexual intercourse every day and don't think it is dangerous. As kissing is regarded as an expression of love rather than a transaction, it is rarely seen in sex transactions. According to our survey, nearly 90% of the "street girls" never kiss whoremasters during sex transactions, so they think that the rare ones are more dangerous. This is actually easy to understand. For example, you drink water every day, but you rarely pay attention whether the water is sanitary. However, if you are suddenly given a weird thing to eat, you will probably check it immediately. What is it? Is it clean? It's a very common psychology.

This means that when doing publicity and education work, we must first know what they already know, which perceptions are wrong, and how we can prescribe the right medicine.

3.5.5 How Do We Get to Know Them?

(1) Believe that I am equal to them

Whether we are doing sociological surveys or doing AIDS prevention work for "street girls", we must have the awareness of "occupation and role cannot be unified", otherwise it will be impossible to approach them, and the or prevention work will have no effect. I have repeatedly emphasized in several of my books that I never go to underground sex trading venues to investigate "street girls", but so far, almost all public health and preventive medicine reports I have read on the "sex industry" came from those places.

In fact, as long as people with a little common sense of life can understand the following things: First, when a saleswoman sells things in a store, it is absolutely different from when she returns home. No matter how thorough your is when she is working, you can only learn a little of her, and it's possible that what you know about her is distorted; Second, since "street girls" regard sex trading as their profession, she must obey the requirements of this "profession" under trading situation. If you investigate when she is at work, how can she say anything? We won't interview the police when he is directing the traffic, so don't "annoy" the "street girls" when she works.

For "street girls" no matter what kind of organization they are in, no matter how equal the sociologists or medical workers treat them, they still regard the later as men of the upper class, and will never completely trust them. This also happens to me when I was doing my research. But under the free employment system and self-management system, the gap is much smaller. They are more confident and think "I am equal to you", so these "street girls" may still be in normal contact and are willing to cooperate with our AIDS prevention work.

This is related to the investigators' genders of the underground "sex industry". In fact, the key lies in the purpose of the. If you just want to skim the surface or investigate superficial issues such as condom use, then male and female investigators are the same and there is no significant difference. Because for the "street girls", these circumstances are not worth being hidden at all. However, if it comes down to personal life and emotion, like whether the "street girls" have any skills to resist sexual assault of whoremasters, they will never tell a male interviewer the truth, because they don't trust any man. The longer they work as "street girls", the less likely they will say anything about your question; however, you just have to get the information you need from such a long-term "street girl".

But when the female students in our institute went out to do a survey, I found the larger problem is that the class gap between women is bigger than that between men and women. The discrimination of good women against bad women is far greater than that of ordinary men. Especially, even if you really don't discriminate against the "street girls", but because they don't think of themselves as bad women, it's difficult to establish an equal relationship if you show characters of good women.

Yan Yuelian, head of Wisteria Organization in Hong Kong, started working as a female worker at the age of 15, then opted for a career in social work for female workers at the age of 19, later engaged in social work for "street girls". Summarizing her years of experience, she said that if intellectual women want to go deep into "street girls" and to be completely trusted, the only way is to "degenerate themselves". Whether they are engaged in AIDS prevention work or doing social surveys, it is not for them to really go into prostitution, but to put themselves in a position equal to "street girls".

This is easy to say but difficult to do. Once a middle-aged female investigator went to a "red light district" with me. After arriving at the residence of a "street girl", she walked around the house, and then stood there for the entire conversation. Even as a man, I felt that: She thought the miss's bed was dirty and didn't want to sit on it. In that way, what is the meaning of telling a "street girl" to prevent AIDS? She believed the "street girl" was just a little girl from the countryside, having no knowledge and no education. Can't that "street girl" know this? In fact, they are more sensitive!

There is also the problem of gender and age. When I went to the "Red Light District" to do surveys or interview the "street girls", I always appeared in the image of their father or even grandfather. They also treated me as one of the old people, not as a man anymore. This diluted their gender awareness and made them less defensive about my interviews. Conversely, when you promised that you are a perfect gentleman and always asked me to investigate with you in the "red light district", you ignored a problem. If you were only in your 20s or 30s, and were so attractive, when a "street girl" loses her heart to you, what were you going to do? It's a very real problem. Once you at least treated them equally, a "street girl" would fall in love with you easily. But all the men who volunteered to follow me to do s about underground "sex industry" had never considered this possibility. If a "street girl" was in love with you, might you love her? Could you marry her? Wasn't your deceiving her feelings? Then what would you do? If you never thought about it, how could I take you there?

(2) Go into their lives

The of the "street girls" must be made in their residences when they are free rather than in the "trading" place when they are working. We should conduct individual consultations instead of classroom lectures and go there with the gynecologist. After that we must issue training certificates.

When doing AIDS publicity and education work, we must bear in mind that the most important thing is not medical knowledge, but: first, the local incidence rate; second, the incidence rate in this circle. Only these two knowledges can directly affect each other's specific behavior.

In addition, we must also pay attention to the latest developments and changes in the underground "sex industry". In many entertainment venues above the mid-range, "sex" of fashionable men has undergone great changes: more flirting; more ways of service; willing to enjoy "non-penetration" sex; taking penetration as the last step of the entire sexual process; don't care about weather wearing a condom or not, hoping to delay ejaculation.

Therefore, our publicity and education work should also change accordingly: we must fully publicize that wearing a condom can increase sexual pleasure, prolong the time of sexual intercourse, alleviate the problem of "vaginal relaxation", and makes the "street girls" more enthusiastic when providing services. In other words, we should no longer use words like "you will die if you don't wear a condom" to scare men.

(3) Education and research must be exchanged

When carrying out AIDS prevention work, we must not have the idea of "I am a doctor, and I will treat you", because we are only helping them to prevent, not compulsorily indoctrinate them. According to the social exchange theory, interpersonal relationships are mainly maintained by exchange, including various non-material exchanges, as well as emotional exchanges. In addition, there are two principles: one is that the exchange must not only be needed by both parties, but also be an equal and fair transaction between these two parties; the other is that if the party with more resources uses its power excessively, it will destroy the exchange between these two parties. As we hope them cooperate with us in AIDS prevention work, we must think about what we should exchange with them? How can it be more equal and independent of authority?

Public health scholars like to use the term "intervention", which is in itself a violation of personal rights. What qualifications and rights do we have to "interfere" with them? We are nothing more than emphasizing that our intervention is for their health and interest, we are here to save them. This idea of "others need me to save" is not based on two equal people. Any two people in society are equal. Under this premise, both parties should change fairly, so that interpersonal relationships can be formed and maintained.

From the perspective of social exchange theory, all social surveys are unequal exchanges. You ask a person about his family size and per capita income, but have you told him your information? In daily life, who can bear such a friend who asks "how much money do you have in your pocket" at the sight of you? If you ask rhetorically, "how much money do you have?" He says, "I won't tell you". In this case, can the friendship between you two go on? Therefore, when you do a survey, you are actually begging the other people to cooperate with you, so never should you hold a condescending attitude. The first lesson in my "Sociology of Sexuality" course was about this: What actually you do when you did a survey? You are begging. It must be such an attitude, and you should never "extort a confession".

If you investigate condescendingly, all the data is basically untrue. Westerners are relatively independent and value the right of privacy. Therefore, there is often a rejection rate of more than 20% in the results of social surveys. The remaining 70% of the respondents are willing to answer, so their probability of answering the real situation increases directly. However, the general personalities of us Chinese are quite different. The Chinese people are "other-directed", not self-oriented. We are not very clear at refusing, but good at disguising and concealing, and even good at lying. Now there are many social surveys, often with a response rate of almost 100%. How can this be believed? For example, though I don't want to talk about my monthly income, I have to say a number at will to dodge you when you insist on asking, and I'm embarrassed to refuse you. For thousands of years, Chinese people haven't been in a society that can fully express themselves. Now all social s are to inquire the specific situation of individuals. The two are inherently contradictory. So now such a simple and crude method of social is bound to force others, and it is definitely using fake data for real calculations.

Especially for disadvantaged groups like "street girl", no matter how interviewers get in touch with them, they still think that interviewers come from the upper class and are different from them. Even if they are willing to be interviewed, they often follow the interviewers' words, which makes it difficult to identify the authenticity of what they said. In fact, we can design the questionnaire in reverse, and let the interviewee comment on something, then the effect will be much better.

3.5.6 They Are the Primary Subjects, While We Are the Secondary Auxiliaries

(1) The top priority: don't get in the way

So what differences our interventions will make in preventing AIDS? I have been a pessimist: the power of man is small. Even if you have interviewed 1,000 "misses" (street girls) and done the "intervention" required, only a few of them who have had real needs accept your work actually. They suspected they were sick or heard some stories of sexually transmitted disease. In a word, they are more enlightened.

Conversely, how can those whose interest were directly harmed by your intervention accept the publicity? How can the boss of entertainment place not hate your AIDS prevention board, which is put in front of the door and causes the loss of customers. The street girl accepts your publicity to use condoms, but she is arrested by police. Condoms become evidence of prostitution. Will she accept your intervention again? Especially for those who don't care their lives, how can they listen to you? They would say, I can live for years although having gotten AIDS, I have had no hope now. Do you care?

Please note that those self-employed street girls are disgusted mostly with the intervention of outsiders. Their consciousnesses are much higher than ours and their reasons, if underestimated, could overwhelm you. They have regarded themselves as normal workers and probably know more than you, but you make "intervention". Will your interventions work well?

(2) We should put ourselves in others' shoes

Most intervention plans I've seen aim to distribute brochures. Actually, it is useless. I specially brought some when I first went to the "red-light district" (this term first appeared in the US in the 1890s when prostitutes placed red lights by their windows to attract customers. Now it refers to an area where prostitution is the main industry.) to do surveys in 1998, but only to find that no one had a look.

Then, I understood that for those low-educated women under "sexual industry", they read nothing, unlike we bookman, taking interest in everything with words. Later, an admirable doctor, who hoped to do something for street girls sincerely, compiled some picture albums of AIDS prevention specially. But I was dumbfounded at the first sight. It was sextodecimo and became octavo if opened further. Where the street girl put it? She sits at the karaoke's bar just with a 32-mo purse. Where she put such a big book? There is no place, except the toilet. What's more, is it possible for her to earn money seeing such a book when whoremaster picks his prey less than a meter away? Why design this? Printing and distributing thousands of such book isn't putting ourselves in others' shoes.

We must enhance mutual understanding to know their following needs when we do intervention. First, the earning. Next, the security. Not arrested by police, not beat up by boss and not raped by whoremaster. Third, confidentiality. Not known by anyone who has relation to them. Usually the last one is to prevent AIDS, because they regard it as a "necessary cost", or most of them have known it enough.

Unfortunately, our current education of AIDS prevention does not consider these things and just requires street girls to do like Lei Feng who sacrificed his individual benefit for the common good, to prevent AIDS for others, to wear condoms in order to avoid the transmission of STD or to do regular jobs. These won't work.

(3) What we should do to help them?

Their first consideration, of course, is earnings. In Europe, AIDS prevention workers will teach street girls the way to earn more money firstly. The more money is earned, the higher positivity of prevention will be. Of course, this has little possibility in China. But, is it hopeless even without 1% possibility? Many street girls don't know how to retain whoremasters or let them pay more, so it is certain that they don't know how to force whoremasters to use condoms. If you're going to teach these low-educated, young girls the way to protect them and deal with whoremasters, you can tell them some psychological characteristics of males, such as what's a good street girl in their minds and how to deal with it and so on. In this way, it is possible to bargain with whoremasters. And the expected effect comes out although we don't directly encourage them to use condoms or teach any specific skills. Moreover, we don't give support to their "businesses" or violate any laws and ethics.

Ostensibly, it may have no relation to AIDS prevention by teaching such things. But in fact, it aims to increase the possibility of using condoms through the improvement of their ability to confront whoremasters. Objectively, it helps to increase their incomes, add understanding and support to our prevention work. When I did survey in Guangdong, I just sat in a hair salon. Many whoremasters, like those who were willing to eat in a popular restaurant, didn't come in if there were just few customers. But when they saw even me, the old man, sat there, they also came in. I didn't violate any laws or morality and just sat there, but there was no doubt that I actually made some helps. Of course, street girls understood what I did and were willing to tell me the truth.

In short, what we should do firstly is to help them build self-confidence so that their basic needs can be met, including active AIDS prevention. When the Wisteria in Hong Kong do prevention, they will discuss a question firstly: is it sincere to do sexual work? If the street girl wants a change, they will offer vocational training and a new job. If she thinks she is suitable to do this without any psychological barriers, they will teach her how to be paid more.

Some girls who do sexual work are young and confused about their lives and futures. They even don't know whether it is a real willingness to do this job when being asked. The pros and cons of all aspects should be told in order to have a clear understanding. After their choices being made, we will help to meet their basic needs, including income, security, confidentiality and others. The last one is AIDS prevention.

(4) Who are the intermediaries

Studies of the "sexual industry" all over the world have found that class gaps between street girls are so wide. Once a street girl rises to a higher level, she will despise those in her original class. The plan our AIDS prevention workers once conceived that asking street girls in higher level to educate those in lower one seems to be impossible.

In this case, AIDS prevention work could only rely on "mommy" (procuress) "chicken head" (pimp) and boss. The first two directly manage street girl at the same status. Usually, procuress is female, pimp male, boss both. The premise, in which they are willing to cooperate with us, is that we do not be a lion in their way to make profits, do not explore their secrets, do not disclose the incidence of AIDS and do not ask ages of street girls. When we arrived at a town in Sichuan, all street girls surveyed on the first day were 18 years old. Is it possible? Later we learned that it was the boss's rule. No matter who asks, you must answer 18 years old because the boss worries being arrested for the employment of children labors. But, the more powerful connection the boss has, the less fear he has and the cooperation with those who once got STD will enjoy a more successful progress.

Currently, our AIDS prevention works should focus on how to "organize and mobilize" boss, procuress, pimp to participate in, because they are the key figures. Having no way to escape, street girls nurture complex emotions toward them. In many cases, they play patriarchal roles as brother and father and order street girls to do this or that. Their words are more effective than our thousands of sentences, and this is the most important feature of the "industry". The similar conclusions haven't been found in western research literatures at present, because of the completely different development of "sexual industry" perhaps. As early as 1995, Chinese Professor Liao Susu and Chinese Professor Wu Zunyou have published related papers about this proposition. However, they didn't attract deserved attentions, because it is impossible for westerners to understand the value of this claim.

3.5.7 The Concept and Model of AIDS Sociology

(1) The concept of AIDS prevention: disease-orientation or people-orientation?

AIDS claims life, but "failed intervention" deprives its meaning.

"Disease-orientation" model is applied in many AIDS intervention plans currently, shown as Fig. 3.7 basically.

This model obviously focuses on sexual behaviors and targets sole individual on the basis of biomedicine. Although it has achieved much, it's still difficult to cope with the "sexualized society" of China in the twenty-first century.

The developing AIDS sociology advocated "people-oriented" model including two perspectives at least. The first one, "the perspective of life ", is shown as the Fig. 3.8. (Please refer to the appendix for more details).

In this model, the individual at risk is no longer a simple organism, but encompasses all aspects of life, and any factor could influence specific choices and actions

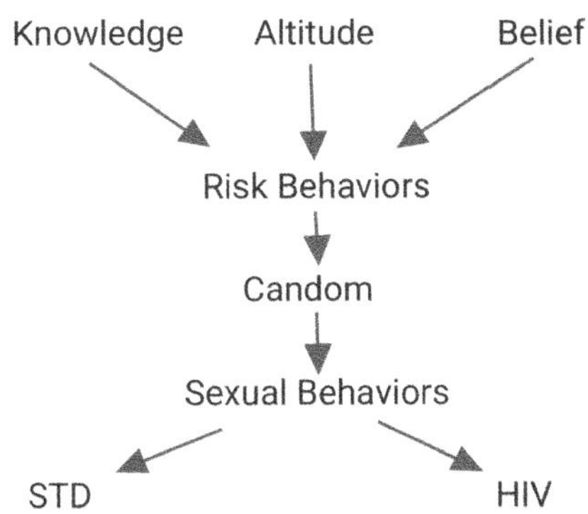

Fig. 3.7 Current AIDS intervention model from "the perspective of communication"

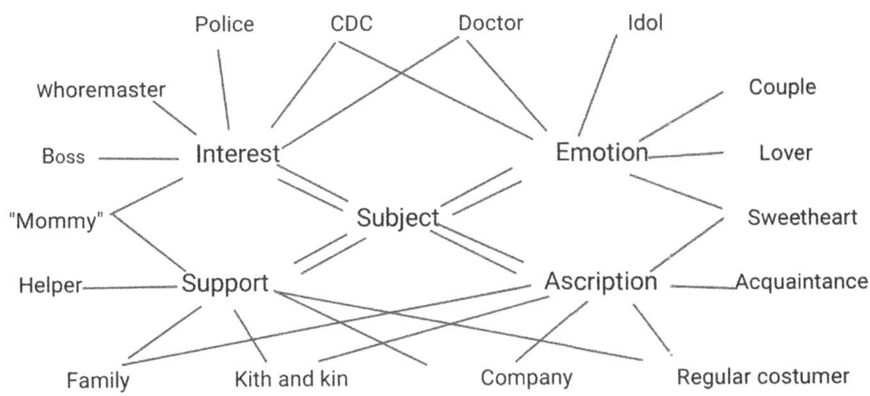

Fig. 3.8 The sociological model of aids from "the perspective of life"

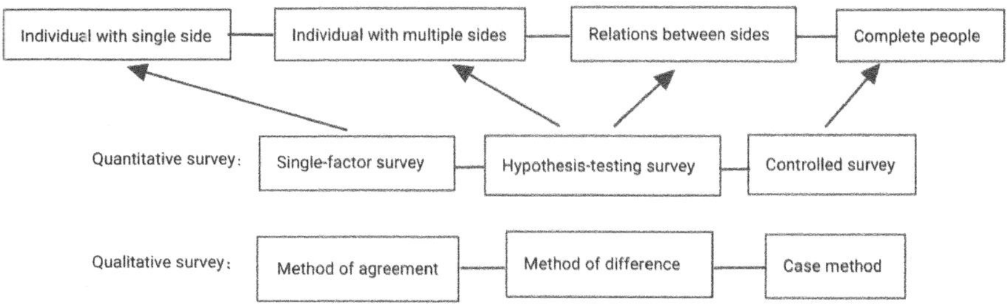

Fig. 3.9 The sociological model of AIDS from "the perspective of communication"

of prevention. In other words, if we do not take a holistic view, prevention work will get half the results with twice the efforts. Thus, the effectiveness will be greatly reduced.

The people-oriented model of AIDS sociology has another perspective, "the perspective of communication", shown as Fig. 3.9.

This model emphasizes that the individual can't live alone in society and all human behaviors are what they are because of various relationships. The same conclusion can also be said for all risk behaviors of AIDS. Therefore, our prevention and intervention work couldn't target one individual, but try to include the whole "interpersonal circle".

(2) The conflicts between AIDS sociology ideas and traditional ones

The conflicts between the ideas of developing AIDS sociology and the traditional ones focus on the following four points.

① Risk bearer: is it the biological people or the social people?

One sentence that advocated by AIDS sociology to treat and advise street girls to cherish their health and life is that: to this world, you are a street girl, but to your loved ones, you are the world.

If such concept is implemented, our intervention work should and could get transformation.

It could gradually transform from the general publicity of "preventing AIDS for all" to "paying attention to the importance of organizational form of 'sexual industry' ".

It could gradually transform from pure medical aspect of "blocking mother-to-child transmission" to "caring about the life of 'prostitute and street girl'".

It could gradually transform from "preventing secondary transmission" to "providing assistance to those who gave up prostitution".

It could gradually transform from the survey of "the ages at which they engaged in 'commercially' sexual actions at the first time" to "the growing pains of women".

It could gradually transform from the determination of the "domicile place" to "seeking marks of hometown".

It could gradually transform from the of "sample sources (classification of places)" to "putting yourself in her small world".

And so on and so forth. All depends on whether our guiding idea conforms to the reality of intervention objects.

1. Risk behaviors: Do they rely on objective detection or subjective construction?

Taking workers as an example, the AIDS sociology argues that transformations from "investigators" to "spokesmen" and from "judges" to "biographers" are necessary. In other words, we should convey subjective cognitions firstly, and then revise our intervention strategies and specific working ways accordingly. Such as:

It could gradually transform from educating "proper use of condoms" to knowing how they "persuade whoremasters to use condoms";

It could gradually transform from forcing them to "work with condoms" to telling them the way of "making next whoremaster more compliant";

It could gradually transform from pure "prevention education" to taking a knowledge of the belief that " I won't be infected";

It could gradually transform from investigating "times of flow" to "summarizing" their "accumulated experience of playing with whoremasters ";

It could gradually transform from focusing on "working frequency" to promoting "skills on psychological and behavioral adjustment" at work.

Only in this way can we achieve the real "peer education" that "encouraging them to share experiences and lessons". Then our interventions will have a clear target and get good results with half efforts.

② Risk group: is it the object of intervention or the subject of right?

The developing sociology of AIDS argues that we should turn the so-called "objects of intervention " into "the holders of rights with the right to health" so as to give a full play to the enthusiasm and initiative of participating in prevention work, which will no longer be regarded as the things that "what I should do" but "what I will do". Such as:

It could gradually transform from treating them as "the main sources of AIDS transmission" to "prominent victims";

It could gradually transform from investigating "the number of sexual workers who don't use condoms" to the surveys of "how many whoremasters don't use";

It could gradually transform from focusing on "the utilization rate of condom" to the number of "street girls" who can "earn same money when they use condoms compared with not";

It could gradually transform from investigating "places they worked in" to ways in which they "develop their interpersonal skills";

It could gradually transform from laying emphasis on the "high-risk sexual behaviors" to popularizing the saying that "persuading whoremasters to wear condoms is the real sexual skill and ability".

Table 3.8 Survey of prostitutes in matteo ricci social services

Working places	Street	Park	Massage shop	Ballroom	KTV
Percentage	63.1%	47.6%	56.1%	69.2%	45.0%
Ages of prostitutes	14–20	21–29	30–39	40–49	50–68
Percentage	42.1	47.4	62.5	63.2	76.3
Working time	Less than 3 months	3 months to 1 year	1 year to 2 years	More than 2 years	
Percentage	25.6	46.8	54.3	73.2	

From 1998 to 2010, I have surveyed street girls in 13 "red-light districts" with my team. What surprised us was that many people had much more knowledge about health and care than average women in many aspects, as well as the awareness, knowledge and capability to prevent AIDS. Actually it is not an oddity. Street girls are not stupid with rich experiences and knowledge, which were accumulated in sexual work, which layman can't get.

But those are just a small part. We should strive to find such "street girls" in our intervention work and provide sincere help to improve their ability instead of instilling medical knowledge, and then making a full promotion of such practical prevention knowledge.

③ Risks come from street girl or the whoremaster?

It is not enough to define that street girl don't use condoms, but to know that: in many cases, it is whoremaster who refuse to use. For example, a survey of 303 young street girls conducted by Matteo Ricci Social Service in Kunming 2017 found that 56.7% of street girls encountered such situation.

The specific situation is shown as Table 3.8.

From the table, our proposition is self-evident: for researchers, the first task is to "rescue" subject. Only in this way can we make our own indigenous and original contributions.

(3) Starting from the goal

What's the purpose of "intervention"? And we do this with what mindset in what way? These are not only the sociological problems, but also medical problems.

The research perspective and method of sociology can be summarized from the perspective of "livelihood-orientation". Because the meaning of disease for the underclass in China never follows medical standards and judged according to the following four aspects: the degree of obstruction to livelihood, the difficulty of solving problem, the subconsciousness of Traditional Chinese Medicine and the fate. If any disease doesn't reach these levels, it will not be regarded as a "disease", and it is certainly impossible to make prevention.

Such underclass is the subject of our prevention. So, no matter how hard doctors try to popularize, the person still view the transmission of HIV as a "fate" or a "necessary cost." For this, the developing AIDS Sociology advocates (in the case of street girl) a two-level intervention goal.

The highest goal is to upgrade their social statuses and empower them, such as striving for the non-illegalization, strengthening gender sensitivity, assisting the organization of street girls. This is the real value of a non-profit nongovernmental organization of AIDS prevention.

The lowest guideline is to understand and meet their needs firstly using "the theory of social exchange" to intervene. The first need is to ensure income (not to go straight or do like Lei Feng), then to ensure safety (not arrested by police, not raped and maltreated by boss/whoremaster), and the third one is to keep secret (not known by related person). AIDS prevention is often the last one.

The division and determination of the highest and lowest goals are very important to AIDS prevention.

After writing the first three chapters, I regret having not given full expression to my views. The differences between sociology and other disciplines are not only in a set of uinque theories and research objects, but also in the sociology is a discipline that relies on empirical research having a whole set of methodology and operation methods about social.

It certainly includes the methods of qualitative research applied in third chapter. But questionnaire survey is more widely used due to its characteristic of "short-flat-fast" in AIDS prevention. It has been used with high frequency by public health workers in particular. For example, almost every CDC of all countries has used questionnaires to investigate the "high-risk population" of AIDS. Their statistics are regularly published in AIDS-related journals of public health. All show that questionnaire has become the leading research method in AIDS prevention.

Unfortunately, these dissatisfied surveys are likely to mislead decision and weaken the effectiveness of prevention work from the view of sociology. In this case, of course, it lacks specific operation. But more importantly, due to the less in-depth and all-around sociological participation, it gives rise to congenital defects in the design of questionnaires. That is the insufficiency of methodology. Therefore, as a sociologist, it is my duty to discuss the methodology of social in order to do my best to promote the development of AIDS prevention.

Unfortunately, I'm not able to discuss all issues of design and operation about questionnaire in this book. If you need more, please refer to the book *On Methods: Local Practice and Sublimation of Sociological,* which is written by Pan Suiming and Huang Yingying and published by China Renmin University Press in 2011. The first half of the book is devoted to the various operational problems of questionnaire. Although it could only focus on some lacking or rare discussions in domestic literature, as a starting point to attract jade, I hope it will be useful for you.

At the same time, as a sociologist, I believe in interactionism and advocate the perspective of subject construction. So, at the end of this chapter, I will go beyond specific cooperation methods to discuss that at what higher levels, the prevention and treatment of AIDS, which is usually regarded as medical issues, promote the cognition and development of sociology, even the whole social science.

References

Suiming, P. (1999). *Existence and Absurdity: An of China's Underground "Sex Industry* (p. 304). Qunyan Press.

Suiming, P. (2000). *Survival and Experience-A Tracking of a "Red Light District* (p. 606). China Social Science Press.

Suiming, P. (2005). *Hooker: The Right to Work-A Comparative Survey of China's Southeast Coastal and Northeastern Cities*. Dadao Press

Suiming, P., Yingying, H., & Zhenying, L. (2005a). Situation and *Perception- Exploring the Three Red Light Districts in Southwest China*. Wanyou Publishing House.

Suiming, P., Yingying, H., & Jie, W., et al. (2005b). *Presentation and Calibration-Deep Research on China's Hooker*. Wanyou Publishing House.

Suiming, P., & Yingying, H. (2007). *Subjective Construction: Revolution and Local Development Space from the Perspective of Sexual Sociology, Sociological Research*, Issue 3.

Suiming, P., & Yingying H. (2008). *Men's AIDS Risk and Intervention*. Wanyou Publishing House.

Yingying, H., & Suiming, P. (2008). Mobility·Sex·AIDS Prevention and Control-Project Report. Wanyou Publishing House.

Chapter 4
The Methodology of AIDS Sociology

4.1 "Process Control" of AIDS

Questionnaire in social science belongs to the school of scientism within positivism in the sense of methodology. It originates from the imitation of "repeatable experiments under controlled condition", one of the basic research methods of natural science, and then reaches its scientificity. The implement of is to imitate "experiment", and random sampling is to imitate "repetition". Although the two points (with random sampling) have been fully understood in our social science, "under controlled conditions", the element of research method in natural science, is not only confined to the bottom lines, such as uniform content and inquiry, but also lacks enough attention in methodology.

The conclusion, "water boils at 100 degrees Celsius" is based on condition that water is kept under "one certain barometric pressure", clearly explains the meaning of "under controlled condition" required by natural science. If it is tested on the Tibetan Plateau, the result would be different. So, the "process control" mentioned in this chapter is not to design "controlled variables" used in the related analysis of questionnaires, but to design a series of methods to control comprehensively and consistently.

From the perspective of "subject construction" I advocate, the implementation of questionnaire is a process of interpersonal interaction actually. And the data investigated is "subjectival presentation", not the so-called "objective fact". So, the "process control" mentioned in this chapter has no more than two elements: first, more attention should be paid to the collection of data, which is conducive to present or explain subject; second, the researcher should actively guide respondents to fully present themselves in interpersonal interaction.

S. Pan, *The Social Construction of AIDS Issues*, A Sociological View of AIDS,
https://doi.org/10.1007/978-981-16-7519-5_4

4.1.1 Living Environment Control: Comprehensive Study of Point

It is a basic consensus in social science that living environment has a great influence on people's consciousness and behavior. And it is not a new idea that respondents give different answers in different living circumstances. So researchers must pay attention to the environment in order to set scientific premise of "under controlled condition" minimally.

Unfortunately, our academic circle doesn't take this point into consideration when we design questionnaire.

Because of lacking such awareness (rather than a lack of practical methods), almost all questionnaires directly focus on individuals and only inquire related information in our social. For this, it will be difficult to get an accurate picture of the living environment where respondents live in even if using refractometry. As a result, what numerous social investigate are "isolated individuals", whose existence no one admit to. And what the data reflects is a "pyramid" society, rather than our real life.

In order to make up for deficiency, I find a new path using the following two methods.

The first is to design a set of quantitative "living indicators of survey sites" in addition to individual questionnaire. It means an investigator (the group leader usually) is arranged at each final survey site ("residential area" in my cases) to collect local data related to individual s on various aspects of daily life as much as possible in addition to individual survey. Quite many social data published by the National Bureau of Statistics can be used to control living conditions. But for one thing, the statistical departments at grass-root level do not provide or even do not have such data; second, the design of indicators usually doesn't meet the requirements of researchers; third, there's little qualitative information. So, I advocate strongly that researcher should design and collect data by themselves. By this, I could obtain two sets of data about personal situation and the related living environment.

The "survey sites", varying from different survey goals, mainly depends on assumptions the researcher makes according to different levels of the living environment which could influence individual's activities. "Life indicators" also vary from survey goals and they are the most related ones researchers hypothesize about individual's activities reflecting the overall living environment.

In fact, the two aspects also follow general principles of designing questionnaire. More "life indicators" should be designed (21–52 items in "four national surveys" for example) if lacking related research (such as research about "sex"); If the cultural influence (e.g., the folklore) is expected to be greater, the scope of "survey site" needs to be more macroscopic (e.g., urban areas).

However, only using the first method is far from enough. What mentioned in second one is more important to obtain overall qualitative cognition through comprehensive fieldwork and your experience and perception. During the process, researchers (at least the commissioned group leaders) are able to get a clear idea of the living condition. This is the rarity what classic questionnaire lacks.

For example, the related living environment in "sex" is not the matter of words. So the quantitative data of "life indicators of survey site" I assume has few variables related to individuals' sexual activities. However, the qualitative cognition (after transforming into attribute data) I (or the group leader) obtained reveals some surprising correlations. For example, the geographical location of survey site (whether it locates in a noisy downtown), the type of house (whether it is a row of bungalow) and the openness of nearby "red light district" (whether the key members of residents are aware of it). All of these affect residents' sexual situation in survey site significantly. Such qualitative cognitions are not only absent from official data, but also unavailable in the collection of quantitative data, so they have to be collected personally.

To say the least, even if qualitative cannot be carried out and what we do is to collect quantitative data, the most important and valuable thing is not the statistic, but the perceptual harvest during data collection. In this way, the qualitative perception and cognition based on statistics could be obtained and become rare resources of current questionnaire surveys. For example, some goals of qualitative s are not be made blindly but triggered by inspirations gained through the collection of quantitative data.

The two methods are not new things and easy to operate. What's more important is that the perspectives of researchers must gradually move from "individualism" to "holism", from "statistic" to "sociology", from "the sum of individuals" to "the whole is bigger than the sum of parts". With such perspectives, "comprehensive of sites" proposed in this chapter will not only arise at the historic moment, but also is indispensable.

Thus, "living environment control" is sufficient to realize the premise of "controlled condition" during data acquisition. Otherwise, the statistical analysis with a large number of incomparable individuals living in different environments will be less scientific.

4.1.2 The Control of Situation: Stimulating Subject to Present Themselves Fully

In our existing courses, it is a necessary content about how to increase the possibility of answering questions. However, scholars always talk about this from the perspective of questionnaire design and mainly discuss how to design questions and alternative answers much easier and accurate. There are also some discussions from the view of investigators, such as being patient and careful in judgment, etc. The concept, even consciousness of situation and its control, have not appeared in the our social scientific literature.

But any specific questionnaire is occurred in a certain situation from the perspective of subject construction, and it is more important that how subjects, the respondents, present themselves in such situation. Because "When in Rome do as Romans do" is neither a deceit nor a disguise but the norm of human life. Therefore, although the adaptability of questionnaire's content and the quality of investigator are able to be enhanced continuously before the beginning of, the scientific premise of "under controlled condition" cannot be realized and the certainty of the results will get great influence if the whole situation of is not controlled.

The so-called "situation" is based on the inevitable interpersonal communications between investigators and respondents during. And as its connotation, the specific environment in which communication occurs, includes various space-time arrangements as well as the atmosphere and interactive modes of interpersonal relationship, etc.

The so-called "process control" is the arrangement that researcher set up in space-time and interpersonal relationship consciously and actively. Its natures existed not in making works more smooth or convenient but in the wholehearted consideration for respondents to make them feel more relaxed and present themselves fully.

Situation control varies with goals. Generally speaking, researchers, at first, should clearly know what situational factors are most likely to prevent respondents from full participation in surveys.

I would like to briefly share my own practical experience. The four "sexual surveys of Chinese adults" I organized are highly sensitive, so they probably had the most stringent requirements on situation. Choosing several major points to expound is beneficial to this chapter and it will help readers to understand the rest using analogy.

(1) Space-time setting

First, I resolutely refuse classic household survey in such a sensitive, for which I won't criticize more. Although some scholars have found its problem and designed other methods to deal with, they didn't question its feasibility fundamentally. Because it is difficult for Chinese people to tell a stranger (investigator) any unruly or non-mainstream sexual relations in their homes, even if there isn't any other person. And they are much more unlikely to share even well-behaved sexual actions, because the situation that "I am in my own home" is so incongruous with "the talk about sex".

As a countermeasure, I specially set up the link of "invitation" during. That is to make a phone call or send a letter to invite respondents to the "interview room" so as to achieve the psychological effect that "the bird is out of the cage".

Second, I set up a special "interview room" in which are carried out, which means an independent, enclosed place is identified prior to the start of as interview site, and there isn't third party. In "Four National Surveys", the places in residential area and nearby hotels, school classrooms, community rooms were the main selections. In terms of response rate and survey results, it showed no significant differences between nearby hotels, school classrooms and community rooms generally, but the first two got better results in smaller cities. It is mainly because the residents there feel more unfamiliar with hotels and rest houses. Then, such "specialized space-time" prompts respondents to present themselves "more specifically".

Third, I used laptop computer to assist my survey each time, that is, to compile electronic questionnaires. Investigators carried their laptops, then respondents read screen's questionnaires and pressed button to answer questions. The greatest benefit of it is that the "interpersonal conversation" of classic questionnaire survey has been changed into "human-computer interaction", which avoids the widespread concept of hearing no evil on "sexual expression" (Chinese couldn't accept investigator to "talk about sex") and passes through the embarrassing cultural barrier (which respondents think inexpressible) to achieve good results in situation control.

(2) Interpersonal relationship setting

First of all, I stipulate that the people who "invite" respondents and the investigator can't be the same one. Because sometimes the former has to mobilize respondent to take survey personally, so he is likely to get some information about respondent (at least they've seen each other). The principle of anonymity will be destroyed if he carries out the. And the respondents will not able to present themselves relaxed, no matter how many promises investigator makes. Therefore, this rule is to ensure the person that every respondent faces is a stranger. It not only keeps secret, but also creates a situation that "he is a stranger and everything is ok "to reduce psychological pressure.

Secondly, I set up the requirement of "increasing intimacy", which stipulates investigator to act friendly so as to achieve the natural atmosphere of a small conversation.

Finally, I insist that the investigator and the respondent must have same sexes. There has been a heated international debate on the gender of investigator. Although some domestic books have talked about this, no special paper could be retrieved. Some foreign researchers found that the gender of investigator has no influence on results. But I hold opposite view because it is wrong to analyze this problem from survey results. I won't say more there. The reason isn't a mystery but comes from the experience of life: how many women will "talk about sex" with male strangers? And how many "sexual talk with opposite sex" will not be regarded as a stimulus, a risk or even a harassment? As a flexible measure, young women are allowed to investigate old males in some certain cases, but I prohibit men to investigate women absolutely.

(3) Computer technology setting

First, I record the gender, age and the degree of education of each investigator in order to infer the possible role of investigator.

Second, I set up the following function in laptop computer: automatic record of the time of answering every five questions and use it to predict the seriousness of respondents.

By comparing the two kinds of data, I could judge the influence of investigator on the process of (not results) and infer the degree of comprehensive implementation of "space-time setting" and "interpersonal relationship setting". Because of convenient laptop, I could make such analysis immediately after each and adjust space-time and investigator at any time.

In conclusion, the actual effect of situation control is that the respondents are more relaxed (not just because of the better designed questionnaire or the smarter investigator) and I obtained higher response rates in similar sexual surveys in China than in America. In China, people are too shy to talk sex and prefer to do rather than talk. Although the impact of time difference and other factors cannot be ruled out, the response rate of the national random sample of American adults in 1992 was only 56 percent, while the response rates of "Four National Surveys" were between 66.5 and 76.4%.

4.1.3 The Control of Data Quality: Collecting "The Performance of Subject Construction"

In our existing literatures, questionnaire is classified into the category of quantitative research rigidly and arbitrarily and we don't dare to cross the scope. Then the "hidden rules" are caused without any rhyme or reason and become latent dangers in operating tutorial. They stipulate investigator asking nothing except question itself, having no notes and just leaving it alone. This is understandable if it aims to save time and effort, but it is more likely caused by a lack of reference to the guiding idea of qualitative.

From the perspective of subject construction, any answer given by respondent is presented to investigator after being constructed in interpersonal interaction. Although researcher and investigator are unlikely to probe into the constructive process on the spot, the does not take place on Mars, so there must be various clues revealing some information. The key point lies in whether we are aware of this or not. Moreover, the respondents are different and everyone has different degree of construction. Therefore, the added collection of information about "respondent's performance" can help researcher to make a precise judgement.

This is the comprehensive judgement of the nature of survey data, an important part of "process control" and the foundation of questionnaire. People are the people. They can change emotions at any time and a same fact will also have different values and significances to them. Otherwise, natural science could not be applied to the study of man.

Unfortunately, it is one of weaknesses of our theories and practices in questionnaire survey.

In fact, judging data quality is more important for questionnaire than qualitative survey. How can we analyze the data if we couldn't determine whether the statements of respondent are affectations or their real colors.

In my limited practical experience, there are some methods to control data quality. I will choose several major points to expound. Controlling data quality is not and cannot be a lie detector, because if you don't know the truth, how can you tell a lie? For this, I won't say more in this chapter.

First, the gender and age of respondent should be separately recorded during the "invitation" and then given to investigator to verify authenticity. In my practice, the rate of impersonation once reached as high as 6% in a place, but all impostors were detected and screened out. we could also form a copy of original data and compare it with the survey data to find out possible impostors. This aims to determine the property of sample.

Second, we increase records of specific situation at the end of the questionnaire which will be filled out by investigator after the departure of respondent. Such as the type of site in which the survey is carried out; whether someone watches or waits outside; whether the children under or over 10 ages are present; whether the is influenced by external factors; whether interruption happens because of external factors and so on.

Third, it requires investigators to record some basic judgments about respondent at the end of questionnaire. For example, did respondent have a drink? If drunk, how much? Was the respondent nervous or shy? Did respondent say more which was not required? Were there some difficulties? Was the investigator needed to provide help? If so, for what? Which local class respondent belongs to according to his dress and so on. I once set up as many as 12 questions.

Fourth, all respondents are encouraged to make complaint which will be recorded. And it requires investigators to ask further information of those who give special answers or responses.

Fifth, in the questionnaire with "the assistance of laptop computer", some functions can be set to reflect the quality of answers, such as the record of the time for respondent to answer every five questions; whether it needs to play the recording prepared for illiteracy and whether we should open the "help window" and so on. With continuous improvements and enhancement of laptop, I believe we will do better in future, such as recording the track of mouse or the specific situation of answer directly.

The basic principle is that all data collected by questionnaire couldn't be original answers. They will be unconsciously "built" when respondents have interpersonal communications with strange investigators in "interview room". An investigator who has methodological awareness of "subject construction" will understand that the so-called "quality control" is actually to make efforts to collect the data that may reflect the process and mechanism of "construction" in addition to their complaints. For example, it is impossible to assure that a person who has drunk must tell a lie, but it will mark the nature of information by noting that "the person has drunk" for related analysis if necessary. If we statistically treat every quality-controlled variable, it will be easy to get the "degree of quality". Adding it to the overall statistical analysis, you will get mathematical results with more "humanization".

In short, although it is easy to set up and enter these variables in laptop, it has great significance to the survey. In fact, this admits and tries to implement the idea that "is interpersonal interaction" and the perspective of subject construction in questionnaire, then it finally gets close to the controlled conditions of scientific research on human.

4.1.4 Moving Towards Integration: The Methodological Significance of Process Control

The specific designs mentioned above not only control quality and prevent the "calculation with false data", but also vigorously popularize the basic idea of qualitative research represented by the perspective of subject construction in the field of quantitative.

It is mainly manifested in the following five aspects.

First, I regard the questionnaire survey as a common process of interaction between the researcher, investigator and the respondent instead of the unilateral attempt of researcher to explore existing objective facts. Special emphasis is placed on the significance of interpersonal interaction between investigator and respondent of the whole study, which is the basic starting point of the "process control" I propose.

Second, I regard the results of the questionnaire as individual's concrete manifestation in his living environment instead of simple performance. So I argue that it is necessary to increase the control of living environment-community in the questionnaire.

Third, I regard the questionnaire as a process in which respondent presents himself in front of the investigator instead of a mere operation of investigator. Therefore, I especially highlight the control of the situation.

Fourth, I regard "subjectival representation" obtained by investigator as a process of continuous subject construction instead of one certain fact. So I suggest that the quality of the data must be controlled.

Fifth, I do not regard the survey as an objective measure like statistics of national economy but a research method for researchers to make a better understanding about real life, to know people in interpersonal communication and to avoid subjective assumptions in controlling subjective initiative.

Now it is obvious that these perspectives are key requirements and operational starting points of qualitative and methodology. One more significant point in this chapter is that it points out we have ability to do such questionnaire and don't have to go through troubles when do them.

4.1.5 A Spectral Understanding of Sociological Methods

My proposition is based on the methodology.

(1) Different survey methods are the classifications of completeness of respondents' performance actually

First of all, the two poles of "spectral existence" should be determined. One pole is the individual with single side which means that respondent is required to present a certain side to investigator. The other side is the requirement which asks respondent to present him fully. Between two poles, different survey methods actually choose

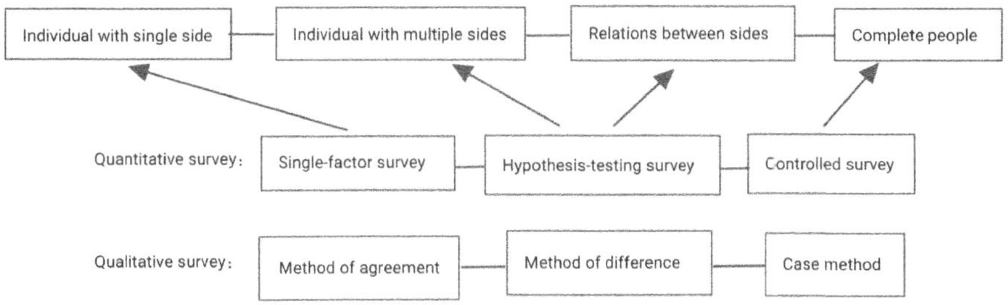

Fig. 4.1 Spectral understanding of survey methods

different domains. For this, I construct the following schematic diagram (shown as the Fig. 4.1).

With such spectral understanding, the essence of "quantity or quality" debate is the different operations for different objectives. Although it's good to use case-study method to investigate whole person, researchers do not need such data but only care about one or more common aspects of respondents in many cases. At this point, they are suitable to be adapted for the objectives no matter the single-factor questionnaire or a qualitative interview with the method of agreement.

But, on the other hand, the distinctions between different survey methods are important as they presuppose and define different domains of spectrum. Our objectives cannot be achieved if we don't investigate the whole people, and any questionnaire methods will ineffective. And if we investigate multilateral relationships between human, neither the single-factor questionnaire nor the qualitative interview with method of agreement can do something.

In this way, the debate of "quantity or quality" turns into a question that what degree should be reached when researcher investigate the "whole person"?

For the questionnaire, the first question is that no matter the lateral aspects, multilateral ones even the multilateral relationship, whether they can be separated from whole "person". And what's the criteria and deviation if they can be separated. For example, in real life, "construction worker" is the stratification of "migrant worker" from the aspect of "the existence of whole person". And it will in vain, if researcher "separates" them from each other and analyzes "construction worker" without considering "migrant worker" or vice versa.

It's a play in mind to define whether aspects can be separated from each other or not. The first thing researchers should do is to demonstrate the rationality and feasibility of any kind of separation. A lack of such awareness is the main problem in our theory and practice of social at present. Although many papers have defined their aspects of, they rarely further explain why this aspect can be separated from the whole and exist in isolation.

At present, the problem also exists in our common qualitative researches of social science. Most of them adopt the method of agreement, which means to research same aspects of people and regard them as examples to prove their analysis and views. But demonstrators rarely discuss that is it impossible to separate "same aspects"

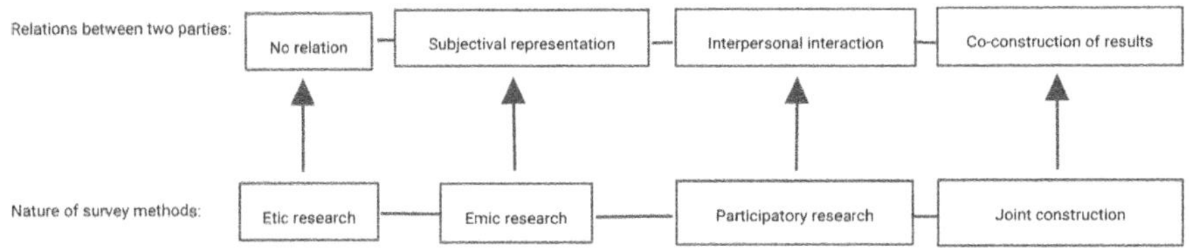

Fig. 4.2 Spectrum of relationship between two parties

from whole. In fact, because of the openness and diffusion of qualitative research, the data listed to prove "they belong to the same aspect" finds that the boundary between aspects is hazy and complex. If demonstrators don't explain these further, it is reasonable to question what's the difference between qualitative surveys from an open questionnaire.

However, in our current methodological discussions, it seems that only qualitative survey emphasizes that we should investigate the "whole person", while the questionnaire survey has no will to learn something from its mistakes and ignores this point deliberately. The main idea of this chapter is to initiate that the process control should be used to get close to the ideal where any social s should reach in.

(2) Relationships between two parties during survey

I can list some spectral existences, shown as the Fig. 4.2.

The meaning of spectrum is that it's far from enough for us to participate in "quantity or quality debate" from the aspect of choosing specific methods. We should analyze the nature of methods from the perspective that "is a kind of interpersonal communication".

As an extreme of spectrum mentioned above, the classical questionnaire usually strictly requires investigators not to induce or influence respondents in order to maintain the objectivity of results. However, as the other extreme, qualitative admits that all results we recorded (including film or television materials) actually influence and construct each other during. Between two extremes, we can intercept certain domains and name them master study, participant study or any other.

Here, as discussed above, the most important thing is not to choose the best but to focus on that whether we have established such spectral understanding, whether we have demonstrated which survey method is consistent with objectives mostly and whether we have made efforts to improve our research in such spectrum.

In this sense, the so-called "quantity or quality" debate does not focus on technical issues that which one are in-depth, meticulous, open and developable but discusses a fundamental question: does interpersonal interaction exist in any one social ? And why do we have to "avoid" or even "ignore" it instead of "controlling" it.

The classic questionnaire seems to a conformist in this aspect. In this chapter, I hope to solve it with "process control".

(3) The integration of vision

Actually, different methods are the different domains which are separated from the same one spectrum, so the "quantity or quality debate" is not a zero-sum game. They can get close even integrate and there is much more room for such development than imagined. In my opinion, each party of the debate demonizes the other unconsciously, which causes more criticisms and less reference then and both of them keep themselves on their own way.

Doubters often give questionnaire the label of "scientism", while people who are questioned are often proud to be "scientific". In fact, it is good to stick to the ideal of "repeatable experiments under controlled condition" in natural science when we study "human". What researchers need is inclusiveness and some perspectives of subject construction to make results in line with the real "person" without making radical changes, let alone kowtowing to qualitative research. In this chapter, I intend to give examples to prove this.

In this chapter, it doesn't mean that "process control" will be achieved only by statistics. Instead, more emphasis is placed on obtaining qualitative experience, perception and cognition in operation. As for the integration of data obtained by the two methods, I believe it is just an icing on the cake rather than a question of paving a way.

Furthermore, such integration is not only at the level of specific methods, but at the integration of guiding idea, research perspective and the soul of the overall design firstly.

Ideally, in such "integrated survey", questionnaire and qualitative survey should learn from each other's strengths to offset weaknesses and make progress together, building harmonious relationship and resolving previous meaningless disputes fundamentally.

I once put forward the proposition of "integration of quantitative and qualitative s". If it's just a proposal, what we do in this chapter is an attempt to discuss its operationalization. As shown in this chapter, after integrating interactive thought into the perspective of subject construction and doing process control, the quantitative researches I carried out have made a small step forward from classical questionnaire to the integration of quality and quantity.

4.2 The Overall Authenticity of the AIDS Survey—A New Method to Verify the Quality of the Questionnaire

In the last chapter we discussed the specific method to carry out the AIDS survey, which may inevitably ignore the general condition. After all what people are concerned about most is the authenticity of the survey results instead of the delicacy of the questionnaire.

Back to 1984 when I was going to step into the field of sociology, once a scholar of another discipline said, "Why do you go to sociology? Sociologists all use false data to conduct study!" These words hurt me but they were motivation to me as well. But during my thirty years of immersion in sociology, I have found that almost none who teaches or study sociology knows what others think of us.

This would be a fatal issue if we were to establish sociology of AIDS. Wouldn't it be such a big crime if we come up with some false or inaccurate data? We might as well not do it! So, to paraphrase someone else's famous saying: even if I have only the last tooth left, I will bite to death "applying false data to conduct study!".

4.2.1 The Difficulty for the Existing Inspection Methods to Verify Authenticity

The authenticity of results is the life of social survey, especially for those sensitive issues. It would be unacceptable for people if the results were lack of inspection and proof to verify its authenticity. The two testing methods mainly adopted domestically are as follows.

The first method is to verify the reliability and validity of the survey. But usually it would be hard to meet its preconditions in two aspects.

Firstly, reliability and validity tests can only be performed on continuous variables, while the main indicators of most social surveys are categorical variables, which are difficult to be converted to continuous variables. Thus, quantitative reliability and validity tests cannot be performed.

Secondly, the premise of performing reliability and validity tests is that all variables to be normally distributed. However, a large number of social survey variables do not meet this premise. The most important variables, such as gender and occupation, are by no means normally distributed. Thus, quantitative reliability and validity tests cannot be performed either.

In particular, the reliability and validity tests can only be performed on the most important variables (usually only one or two variables), which cannot reflect the authenticity of the whole survey.

The second method is to set lie-detecting items in the questionnaire, mainly by using logic tests and repetition tests. But here comes the same problem.

There can't be too many lie-detecting items. Once lie answers appear, the sample can only be deleted, i.e., deleting all the answers of the respondent are required. However, the other answers of the respondent are most likely not lies, as a result, our deletions are likely to be biases and a great loss of the amount of information. Conversely, even passing the lie detection on one or two of the most important.

In brief, the above two methods adopted at present both have the defect of ignoring the general condition. But as for social surveys aimed at sensitive issues, we care most about the authenticity of the whole questionnaire. If the overall authenticity is questioned, none of the results are valid. Unfortunately, reliability and validity tests and lie detection cannot provide us with such information.

Targeting the above problems, I put forward three new testing methods based on my own experience for references. Since it is primarily an introduction to methods, statistical procedures are no longer listed.

What I relied on were the first three stratified equal probability sampling surveys of the total population of China conducted by myself.

4.2.2 Respondents' Self-Answer Design

My first hypothesis is that due to the reasons such as low education level and lack of time, respondents who do not understand the items in the questionnaire are more likely to tell unintentional lies or give wrong answers. Hereby, I designed a specific quiz and put it at.

at the end of the questionnaire. The percentage in the brackets is the statistical analysis of the complex sample.

The survey is coming to an end. We have asked you a lot of questions. Do you understand what we are asking? Do you know the concrete intention of the questions? (N = 17,988).

1. I don't understand most of them (4.2%)
2. I don't understand half of them (8.3%)
3. I understand most of them (48.9%)
4. I understand all of them (38.9%).

My second hypothesis is that the more sensitive the respondents believe the questions in the questionnaire are, the more likely they are to lie. Hereby, I designed a specific quiz as follows (N = 17,908).

Do you find the above questions sensitive to yourself?

1. Very sensitive (17.3%)
2. Kind of sensitive (49.3%)
3. Not too sensitive (23.6%)
4. Not sensitive (9.6%).

The two quizzes above are intended to verify the overall authenticity of the questionnaire from the perspective of the respondents' self-statement.

4.2.3 On-Scene Investigator Monitoring Design

The respondents always answer questions in front of the investigators. Therefore, the on-scene observation of the investigator becomes a valuable objective monitoring. Hereby, I designed a quiz as follows, which was to be filled by the investigator after the respondents left. The numbers in the brackets are the statistical results of the complex sample for your reference.

My hypothesis is that the presence of other people reduces the authenticity of the answer. Hereby, two quizzes about the situation are designed.

Were there children present at the interview? (N = 18,006).

1. Yes (1.1%)
2. No (98.9%).

Were there other people present at the interview? (N = 18,006).

1. Yes (1.1%)
2. No (98.9%).

My hypothesis is that the respondents who need to be mobilized again, who need a lot of help and who drink alcohol will be less truthful. Hereby, four quizzes about the investigators' observation are designed.

Whether the respondents need to be mobilized again during the ? (N = 17,989).

1. Much needed (1.4%).
2. Barely needed (54.7%).
3. Not needed (43.9%).

How much help do the respondents need when answering the questionnaire? (N = 17,949).

1. Often needed (11.6%).
2. Sometimes needed (15.3%).
3. Barely needed (17.7%).
4. Not needed. (55.4%).

Did the respondents drink wine when they came? (N = 17,953).

1. A lot (0.6%).
2. A little (5.5%).
3. Didn't drink (93.9%).

According to your observation, were the respondents honest? (N = 17,550).

1. Very dishonest (0.5%).
2. Less honest (7.2%).
3. More honest (57.7%).
4. Very honest (34.6%).

All the above six quizzes can be used as the basis to estimate the overall authenticity of the respondents' answers.

4.2.4 Design for Answer-Time-Based Testification

The was performed through notebook computer, namely, every item was presented at the screen and we asked the respondents to answer the questions by pressing number buttons. This method is the best practice for sensitive s which is adopted internationally and in itself helps to increase the proportion of authentic answers.

Besides, another advantage of this method is that it can secretly record the time every respondent costs when answering the questions. And according to the number of questions answered, the average time to answer each question can be calculated.

My hypothesis is that outside a certain interval of the average answering time, the shorter it is, the less serious the respondents are. Conversely, the longer it is, the more likely the respondents to be indecisive or unable to understand the questions.

Both conditions will increase the probability of lie answers or wrong answers. Hereby, I take the average answer time as one of the methods to verify the authenticity of the whole questionnaire.

In the Fourth National Survey, based on the number of questions answered, the average time cost of each question was 1.81 min (standard deviation = 1.07; mean standard error = 0.012). With such a new variable, we can use a variety of statistical methods to process the data in order to estimate the earnestness of the sample responses from the answer time.

4.2.5 *The Determination and Significance of Overall Authenticity*

As is stated above, the method we adopt above will gain us a total number of nine variables from three aspects (comprehension and sensitivity of self-statement, six variables from field monitoring and the average answer time). We can then use a variety of statistical methods to come up with a comprehensive overall authentic variable. The concrete steps I take are as follows. First, each variable was processed into "Yes" and "No" (0 and 1), and then factor analysis was used to obtain the factor value with a cumulative interpretation rate of 55.88%. Such is the measure result of the overall authenticity of each sample.

No matter what statistical method is used, we can always obtain a quantitative variable to mark the overall authenticity according to the train thought above. In the subsequent further statistical analysis, as long as this authenticity variable is included in the analysis, either as a weighted number or as a control variable, we can modify the authenticity of the analysis results to maximally approach the real situation.

The improvement of this method compared with the reliability and validity tests is that it can be applied to the most common categorical findings in social surveys, which is vivid and easy to explain. Its improvement over the polygraph test method is that it does not need to delete certain samples, but it can control the degree of inauthenticity.

Most importantly, the reliability and validity test and lie-detecting test can only be applied to the main variables of the questionnaire while my new method can reflect the overall authenticity of the survey. Furthermore, it provides not just the judgement of "true or false", but a qualified "degree" which can be statistically calculated.

I sincerely hope that all of the above will contribute to the advancement of social survey methods.

4.3 Combination of Sociology and Public Health: Discussion of Incidence of AIDS

Worldwide, long-term and repeated studies have found a significant positive correlation between HIV infection rates and the incidence of STDs. Therefore, many countries or regions use the incidence of STDs to make the corresponding judgment on the spread of AIDS due to the difficulty of popularizing HIV tests.

Therefore, we will discuss the incidence of STDs in this chapter. However, this discussion is not purely statistics but an attempt to provide an instance to show how sociological research and public health work are combined.

At present in China, all the information about the incidence of STDs in the total population, whether the proportion of infected people or the proportion of people who develop sexually transmitted diseases, is obtained by using the method of testing, i.e., summarizing the data of medical testing at different monitoring points across the country. This method has been internationally used for hundreds of years, and its accuracy seems impeccable. But the sociological "incidence" of all phenomena, including diseases, is determined by social survey with strict random sampling.

Thus, two sets of data of STDs appear. Although health institutions and their highest authorities in our country have always trusted only the monitoring data of their own departments, such two sets of data will sooner or later arouse social controversy with the great development of sociology and the popularization of social survey. We should take precautions, so we must discuss it in this book.

4.3.1 Why to Need Self-Reported Incidence

In this section, I use data from the Fourth National Survey for a sociological analysis to deepen and expand our understanding of the mechanisms underlying the incidence of STDs.

In our questionnaire we asked the following questions: "Currently in China, many people have been infected with social diseases, and have you ever been diagnosed with such disease so far as gonorrhea, syphilis, acute eczema, genital herpes and non-gonococcal urethritis?".

The first sentence of the question may be regarded as an induction, but in today's China, there is still a strong moral stigma against STDs. Hence, it is necessary to use that sentence to reassure the interviewees. Meanwhile, my hypothesis is that people won't exaggerate the incidence of STDs due to the moral stigma.

The use of the term "social diseases" rather than the standard statement "sexually transmitted disease" (STD) is due to the fact that a total population survey requires the use of terms that low-educated population can understand.

The original phrase "been diagnosed with social diseases" was expressed in the questionnaire of the Fourth National Survey as "did a doctor in a regular hospital tell you that you have social diseases".

However, in my subsequent quantitative I found that, many street girls and whore-masters (johns) go to private clinics instead of regular hospitals. Therefore, such statement will leave out the incidence of STDs.

In short, self-reported STD incidence is clearly not equivalent to prevalence rate. This index is investigated and analyzed mainly because of the following three reasons.

First, it can be used for the general population survey to be nationally representative, especially for STD patients who do not go to any health care provider at all but take medication by themselves. There should be some functional relationship between it and the actual prevalence.

Second, because my questionnaire basically covers all aspects of Chinese people's social stratification and sexual relation and behavior, the phenomenon of self-reported.

STDs can be put in a broader framework and analyzed from more perspectives.

Third, self-reported STD exposure is in itself a sign of STD awareness and coping strategies. The most likely situation is that if they do not know that they have STDs, the possibility of people taking the initiative to examine STDs will be greatly reduced, much less likely to take the initiative to learn about the prevention knowledge of STDs. Therefore, investigating the incidence of self-reported STDs will help us to carry out STD prevention work more effectively.

None of these above three academic implications can be realized in the current survey of the STD prevalence in China, which relies on outpatient reporting and sentinel surveillance. The discussion in this section is therefore intended to fill in the gap rather than replace the prevalence rate.

4.3.2 *The of the Commonalities of Each Historical*

There are two major deficiencies in the present STD statistics based on public health theory.

The first is to focus only on development tendency of the incidence of STDs, and to use the incidence by year as a separate number. But we all know with common sense that the infection of STDs is the result of the continuous accumulation of multiple partner sexual behaviors over a long period of time, and accidental infection of STDs is actually rare. As a result, the annual statistics of public health cannot measure the incidence and development of STDs from the perspective of a historical period.

Secondly, the uniqueness of STDs is that their incidence is closely related to social and cultural changes in a given historical period rather than being simple diseases in biological sense. However, the current statistical methods of public health cannot reveal the content of this aspect, let alone explain its significance.

For that reason, I would like to show what long-term, economic and cultural factors can be found to significantly influence the incidence of STDs in China through the results of strict random sampling survey in sociology.

(1) **Social class analysis of male STDs: The "irrational" aspects and their implications**

The Fourth National Survey used basically the same questionnaire, which could be divided into 10 different fields. Firstly, the factors significantly correlated to the occurrence of STDs in various fields were examined, and then regression analysis in all fields was conducted. To save space, the complex statistical process is not listed.

① The incidence of STDs not higher among younger people, but among men in their 30s.

Men aged 30–34 are the most likely to get STDs, more than 200 times than the national published data. Men aged 35–44 is the second most likely group, while the youngest men aged 20–24 are the least likely.

The reason is that STDs are most likely to be transmitted by sexual behavior of multiple partners, but males under 25 are not yet able to devote a large proportion of their time to it due to their lack of social experience. Meanwhile, men over 45 are lack of competitive advantage and drive, so the middle age group of men stands out. Especially, most men of this age group are newly married and have young children, so for them STDs are not a simple morbid problem, but a problem with strong social significance for marriage and family.

This kind of circumstance also reminds us that, at present the propaganda education to prevent STDs and AIDS has a "younger age" trend day by day, paying more and more attention to adolescents but inclining to ignore those men who become fathers and husbands. This is not a kind of distracted trend, but also not conductive to the prevention of secondary transmission of STDs between husbands and wives.

② STDs not the most prevalent among the floating population but the opposite.

That is because the life of the migrant population in the inflow region often has three main characteristics as follows.

Firstly, they are unfamiliar with the inflow regions, aimless and relatively lacking in the ability to find partners necessary for multiple sexual behaviors. And it may take them a long time to find where to go even for prostitution.

Secondly, they have almost no "freedom of local social intercourse". In addition to their busy work and lack of spare time, they don't want to go out either because they don't fit in with the city or are closed off by work.

Thirdly, they also often lack cash-paying capacity, for many migrant workers only get one-off paid when they return home at the end of the year. In other words, even if they want to go whoring in spare time, they could not pay with "IOUs".

In particular, there are also huge differences among the migrant population. The migrant population that can break through the above three restrictions is definitely not those fully or partially enclosed migrant workers in the factories or on construction sites but those who work in small shops, open fairs, auto parts cities and home decoration stores where many rural migrants congregate.

By contrast, local males, even if they are good for nothing, tend to innately or more easily to break though all three of the above limitations.

This suggests that rather than targeting migrant workers to prevent STDs and AIDS, we should go into local communities and directly educate local males.

③ The incidence of STDs the least among those highest and lowest educated people.

This may be that men with intermediate levels of education, such as middle and high school education, are capable enough to increase their confidence, ability and opportunities to engage in multiple partner sex, but at the same time are not constrained by ambitious goals. Therefore, they have the highest continuous accumulation ratio of infecting STDs.

Conversely, men with junior college education or above may have better conditions in all aspects, but they tend to receive more constraints.

The first is that "love worship" makes them less likely to go whoring; second, the requirement of "perfect matches" makes them less likely to visit prostitutes or have one-night stands; the third reason is that they tend to be ambitious and less willing to have multiple partner sexual behavior encumber their prospects. As a result, they have a lower incidence of STDs.

Those with the lowest education are likely to be acutely aware of the fact that they are in the most disadvantaged position in society in every way. Any kind of multi-partner sex is much less likely to appear among them either by not acting on their own will or by not being able to do anything about it. Consequently, the incidence of STDs are accordingly lower.

④ STDs being "illness of affluence".

As the folk says, the incidence of STDs is related to "the man becomes corrupted when he has money". According to the Fourth National Survey, STD incidence rates are the lowest among the 40% men with the lowest income; slightly higher among the 30% men with middle income; roughly average among the 20% man with higher income, yet the highest among men with the highest income, more than a hundred times higher than the national average for the whole population.

So, which of the above social class factors plays the most important role? Or, when it comes to STD prevention, which group of men should we target most? This requires regression analysis with the self-reported incidence of STDs as the target variable. The analysis results of the 2010 survey are shown in Table 4.1.

Table 4.1 clearly shows that income is the only factor significantly associated with the occurrence of STDs. That is to say, if we really want to prevent STDs, we should first and mainly carry out publicity and education through tax bureau for those who earn more than 120,000 yuan a year and have to pay individual income tax alone, rather than for those of low income, low age, low education and non-local household registration.

Table 4.1 Logistic regression analysis of the incidence of self-reported STDs in men and their social class

Variable name	B	S.E	Wald	df	Sig	Exp (B)
Average monthly income	0.660	0.195	11.454	1	0.001	1.935
Years of education	0.137	0.050	7.580	1	0.006	1.146
Local residents or not	0.239	0.093	6.660	1	0.010	1.271
Live in the county	−0.604	0.301	4.036	1	0.045	0.547
Live in the city	−0.531	0.333	2.541	1	0.111	0.588
Live in provincial capitals, municipalities	−0.499	0.381	1.710	1	0.191	0.607
Occupation and social status	−0.055	0.054	1.022	1	0.312	0.947
Party members or not	0.170	0.288	0.349	1	0.554	1.186
Control variable: year of survey	−0.213	0.227	0.883	1	0.347	0.808
Control variable: age	−0.008	0.011	0.471	1	0.492	0.992
(Constant)	−5.738	1.015	31.939	1	0.000	0.003

From this perspective, the social meaning of STDs and AIDS is definitely not only the influence it has brought to society, but what kind of people that the prevention of STD and AIDS has influenced.

Besides those engage in prostitution, the present prevention work of China is precisely aimed at the disadvantaged groups in society. For example, by 2010, if you search "the prevention of STDs and AIDS+XXX" in Google China, there are 81,900 results of teenagers, 59,800 results of undergraduates, 19,900 results of rural migrant workers, even 12,400 results of long-distance truck drivers. This shows that these issues are highly appreciated in China. On the contrary, there are only 12,300 results of STD and AIDS prevention targeting high-income people, 7960 for high-income people, and only 2900 for income difference.

In brief, in present China the prevention work of STDs and AIDS miss the target group and add much mental pressure to those disadvantaged social group. To some extent, it is even stigmatization. This originates not only from the deep-rooted awareness of "grassroots" and "pariahs" in our tradition, but also the interest orientation brought by the intensified social stratification in recent years.

(2) **Female STDs: The embodiment of the disadvantaged position in marriage**

First of all, the logistic regression analysis of social stratification of women surprisingly reveals that the self-reported incidence of STDs in women was only significantly correlated with her overall health condition, not with any other major personal health indicators of herself, even her own multi-partner sex. See Table 4.2 for details.

So, are Chinese women's STDs appearing out of nowhere? The regression analysis of all data demonstrates that almost all factors significantly related to female STDs come from their marriage and the condition of their husbands.

It was impossible for us to know whether a woman's STD was transmitted by her husband because our survey did not ask spouses. But we were able to analyze the conditions of those husbands whose wives had been infected with STDs.

Table 4.2 Logistic regression analysis of the incidence of self-reported STDs in women and their personal indicators

Variable name	B	S.E	Wald	Sig	Exp(B)
Overall health condition	0.564	0.185	9.269	0.002	1.758
Number of sexual partners for more than one month	0.734	0.341	4.622	0.032	2.083
Smoking frequency	0.706	0.347	4.141	0.042	2.027
Live in the city	0.778	0.450	2.991	0.084	2.177
Total number of sexual partner last annual	0.439	0.330	1.770	0.183	1.551
Local residents or not	0.166	0.141	1.384	0.239	1.181
Living in the county	−0.569	0.568	1.002	0.317	0.566
Tendency to lose weight	−0.354	0.375	0.891	0.345	0.702
Party members or not	0.589	0.630	0.876	0.349	1.802
Degree of obesity	0.284	0.356	0.637	0.425	1.328
Years of education	0.051	0.065	0.613	0.434	1.052
Total number of sexual partners	−0.259	0.434	0.357	0.550	0.772
Live in provincial capitals, municipalities	−0.347	0.689	0.253	0.615	0.707
Monthly average income	0.131	0.338	0.151	0.698	1.140
Degree of self-attractiveness	0.073	0.263	0.077	0.782	1.075
Occupation and social status	−0.027	0.103	0.068	0.794	0.973
Drinking frequency	−0.008	0.355	0.001	0.981	0.992
Control variable: year of survey	1.565	0.749	4.365	0.037	4.784
Control variable: age	0.002	0.020	0.007	0.933	1.002
(Constant)	−12.345	2.458	25.225	0.000	0.000

The omitted cross table shows that if the wife's family is better off than the husband's, only 0.7% of the wives have STDs, but if the husband's family is better off than the wife's, 2.5% of the wives have STDs.

Similarly, if there are conflicts between husbands and wives and the husbands' families won't back them up, then the percentage of wives with STDs is just 0.7%. Otherwise, the percentage of wives with STDs is 4.1%.

The same is true in married life. If husbands don't show enough consideration for wives, the incidence of STDs of wives rises from 0.8 to 2.1%.

If wives are being jealous of their husbands, the incidence of STDs of wives rises from 0.5 to 2.3%.

Certainly, if husbands have sexual behavior with others, the incidence of STDs of wives will rise from 0.7 to 3.4%.

In conclusion, those husbands with better conditions, backed up by their families, without giving enough consideration for wives, making their wives jealous and having extramarital sexual behaviors are undoubtedly in the superiority of the power relations. In these marriages, wives are not only the weak sociologically, but also "second-class gender" in the social gender sense. It is this subservery status that has become a related factor in a woman's STDs.

So, which of those are more relevant in the above factors? See Table 4.3 for details.

Table 4.3 Logistic regression analysis of the incidence of self-reported STDs in wives and their marital status

Variable name	B	S.E	Wald	Sig	Exp(B)
Be jealous to husband or not	1.366	0.438	9.719	0.002	3.920
Husbands have extramarital sexual behavior or not	0.959	0.334	8.246	0.004	2.608
Husbands' families back them up or not	−0.561	0.199	7.969	0.005	0.570
Wives have extramarital sexual behavior or not	−1.066	0.401	7.084	0.008	0.344
Husband be jealous to wives or not	−0.831	0.383	4.706	0.030	0.436
Comparison of chore done by husbands and wives	−0.193	0.130	2.192	0.139	0.825
Husbands give enough consideration or not	−0.516	0.354	2.118	0.146	0.597
Husbands' families are better off or not	−0.266	0.196	1.838	0.175	0.766
Degree of affection between husbands and wives	0.158	0.255	0.384	0.535	1.171
Control variable: year of survey	1.271	0.541	5.521	0.019	3.563
Control variable: age of husbands'	0.021	0.017	1.590	0.207	1.021
(Constant)	−3.589	1.720	4.356	0.037	0.028

Table 4.4 Different incidences of self-reported STDs in different relationships

Cases	never	sometimes	Sig	Exp(B)	OR up	OR low
Group sex (last year)	3.0	44.8	0.000	6.253	4.133	9.460
Use of new drugs	4.8	36.3	0.000	3.070	1.927	4.891
Exchange of sexual partner	3.5	25.6	0.000	2.229	1.456	3.413
Once had an affair (accumulated)	2.6	9.7	0.000	2.245	1.655	3.046
One Night Stand (last year)	3.5	12.6	0.000	1.897	1.356	2.654
Once went to sex workers	3.4	20.2	0.006	1.793	1.186	2.711
Prostitution	3.4	21.9	0.071	1.489	0.966	2.294
Once had an affair (last month)	3.8	11.2	0.179	0.584	0.266	1.280
Crossed sexual partners (last year)	5.0	17.2	0.251	0.738	0.439	1.240
Touch the private part of the dancing girl	3.8	16.2	0.287	1.281	0.812	2.019
Private part messaged by opposite sex	3.5	16.6	0.360	1.214	0.801	1.838
Whoredom	3.6	22.3	0.476	1.186	0.743	1.893
New sexual partners (last year)	3.6	11.2	0.563	1.199	0.648	2.218
New sexual partners (last month)	3.9	13.2	0.934	1.030	0.517	2.051
(Constant)			0.000	0.043		

*Control variables: gender, age, level of education, absolute heterosexual or not. Statistics are no longer listed

This clearly indicates that the superior status of husbands and the wives' second-class status are significant factors that influence the incidence of STDs of wives. In particular, even the wives' own extramarital sexual behaviors take a back seat and can't be a significant factor. This well proves the correctness of my inference.

Certainly, none of the above cases is surprising because the high incidence of STDs of wives often results from husbands' multiple-partner sex, especially prostitution. But the question is that in such a socialist country of ours whose Constitution says that men and women are equal, why has this aspect of problems not receiving enough attention until the STDs and AIDS upburst today?

If the wife is infected with STDs by her husband, she is definitely 100% victim of secondary transmission within marriage. Can she then file for divorce and claim for compensation? Why "the crime of propagating STDs" has long existed in our Criminal Law but in the Law on Protection of Rights and Interests of Women and Children, there is no provision to protect the injured wives?

Though this is not the concern of public health workers, it would be very helpful to promote the cause of AIDS prevention objectively if we sociologists offered it to the highest decision-making departments. This can be the best channel of the mutual combination and promotion of the two sides.

4.3.3 Interrelation Between Historical Development and Social Class

Public health study, of course, has never overlooked research in this area, but it still has no advantage over sociological research. Therefore, the following analysis of mine intends to use instances to promote the combination of the two disciplines, and jointly create and improve the new discipline of sociology of AIDS.

The following significant information can be found from statistical analysis of the "Fourth National Survey".

(1) The social stratification of sexual orientation (absolute heterosexual or not) is hard to be observed directly in our daily life or in outpatient reception. But it is not only the most significantly relevant variable, moreover, the percentage of non-heterosexual self-reported STDs has already reached one third, the possibility of which is 21.6 times higher than the absolutely heterosexual.

(2) Although the rate of self-reported STDs in women is similar to that in men, but it was only 64% after expelling other factors which may be influential. This is at least partly because the percentage of non-heterosexual are higher in men.

(3) In the age group under 30, the rate of self-reported STDs is 7.7%. From the age of 18 onwards, the rate of self-reported STDs decreases by 2.6% for every one-year increase in age. This is apparently related to the decrease in sexual activity with age.

(4) The rate of self-reported STDs of the divorced and the widowed is four times higher compared with the married.

(5) The rate of self-reported STDs in people with degree of junior high is 2.9 times compared with those of higher education. The effect of education level on the overall tendency is that the rate of self-reported STDs in low educated people is higher.
(6) The rate of STDs among urban workers of any occupation is significantly higher than that among rural workers. Among them, the proportion of ordinary workers in business service industry, entrepreneurs and leading cadres at all levels is remarkably high, which is 1.8–2.6 times higher than that of other occupations.
(7) There is no significant correlation between the amount of income, the migrant population or not and the possibility of self-reporting STDs.

All the findings of the above study are often seen as purely sociological results. However, if we look at it from a new perspective, in conjunction with public health work, we are fully aware of its significance. Only some potential development directions are listed.

While HIV prevention research and work have already highly focused on the upburst prevalence rate among MSM populations (men who have sex with men), the most important concept MSM still does not cover all people with potential risks. In other words, the "non-absolute heterosexuals" I have surveyed did not necessarily have "male-male sex," but the orientation was almost definite. Hereby, the research on the possibility of HIV transmission will be more prospective if public health research can adopt the new concept of our sociology.

Although AIDS prevention work is not yet able to directly intervene in the risky sexual behavior of all spouses in China, it is entirely possible to have a try on those divorced and widowed according to my research results. This would not add too much work, but would be enough to put the word "prevention" more thoroughly into practice. The others won't be enumerated. Readers can draw inferences from the above case.

4.3.4 Which Sexual Behaviors Are at Higher Risk of STD Infection?

In the prevention work of AIDS, more and more people are beginning to place greater emphasis on the phenomenon of "sexual transmission", but they wrongly see the composition ratio of the internal route of infection as the incidence among the whole population. The result is that the so-called misconception "the possibility of sexual transmission is increasing" spreads more and more widely, it not only misleads the public but also leads to a bias in prevention decisions and main directions.

In fact, the so-called "sexual transmission" includes various channels and involves various sexual behaviors and population. It should not be generalized nor be settled on a single authority. Therefore, the sociological method is used to analyze it, and hopefully it would contribute to the in-depth, detailed and targeted prevention work.

It provides us with important implications as follows.

(1) Sex with highest risk is not the "street girl" sex (it comes only in the sixth place), but mainly non-transactional multi-partner sex between ordinary people. The incidence of these behaviors in the general population is much higher than that of men and women who engage in prostitution. It has played a significant role in putting self-reported STDs at the top of the list.
(2) Hypothesis in the questionnaire is that crossed sexual partners and new sexual partners would increase the chance of STD infection. But this hypothesis has not been confirmed. Neither behavior was significantly associated with the rate of self-reported STDs.

It is also at least a reminder of the following things to be aware of in the Public health can do little, at least for now, about non-transactional, multi-partner sex among ordinary people. Some senior leaders privately admit that prevention work is already under pressure and they don't want more. However, you can do without work, but you can't do without thinking. For example, in order to prevent "sexual transmission", the intervention of underground sex service providers should not only target whether they use condoms or not. This is non-commercial sex, and ignoring it may make our prevention efforts less effective.

4.3.5 Revelation: Objective Measurement is Compatible with the Perspective of Subject Construction

As for the incidence of STDs, biomedicine-based preventive medicine and public health have always insisted on objective measurement. This is, of course, the result of hundreds of years of natural science development, which has brought infinite benefits to mankind.

However, after entering the twenty-first century, more and more people have been infected with STDs non-accidently, non-passively and non-sexually due to their actively choosing to engage in certain high-risk sexual behaviors. As a result, it has brought some issues that must be academically figured out.

The first question is that if those who claims to have STD hasn't had a proper medical test, how on earth do they know they are infected.

Is it because that some symptoms appear on them or they are actually aware that those sexual behaviors they engaged in are of high risk so they become extremely sensitive? Or is it that they feel regretful or guilty of their risky sexual behaviors so they exaggerate their chances of getting STDs?

Here it's not about the issue of their misdeclaration but about the possibility that people's own sexual behavior, the value evaluation and result prediction of this behavior, are only possible after they carry out the "subject construction". Self-reported STD is a good example.

This new perspective is of vital importance to the specific prevention work of STDs and AIDS. Because for those who have already been diagnosed with STDs by medical tests, the problem only lies in treatment and the prevention of secondary transmission. However, the people that our prevention work faces are precisely not such group but those who have been engaged in risky sexual behaviors. Therefore, our research needs to go further, not only to find out what kind of symptoms they had before they thought they were infected with STDs according to medical thinking but also to have an in-depth understanding from the sociological perspective of subject constructure: what kind of significance and value do they give to all kinds of sexual behaviors? And how do they predict the consequences of these sexual behaviors? In particular, what are the ongoing consideration and choices they make between risky sexual behavior and the possibility of infecting STDs? How is this process implemented or interrupted?

All the above research from the new perspective is actually providing us with a new path in our prevention work besides effective medical testing, and finally reaches a better condition of double-track system.

4.4 New Perspective AIDS Has Brought to Sociology

In the previous part of this book, the author highlighted the participation and promotion of prevention in public health from the perspective of sociology. But on the contrary, the research and specific work in prevention of AIDS also have a huge impact on the field of sociology.

It is not only an opportunity to "hitch a ride on AIDS", but also a challenge to many existing sociological research results. This has forced us to establish some new perspectives, first and foremost not to participate in disease prevention, but to develop our discipline. Unfortunately, many scholars in the sociological field have not yet realized this point, and may still regard the emerging sociology of AIDS as a "side issues". Therefore, this chapter is mainly addressed to my colleagues in sociology.

4.4.1 How Individuals Organized to Exist and Participate in Society?

In the process of studying AIDS internationally, the unit of measurement for those who have high-risk behavior to get AIDS are at first called "person" or "people". And nowadays the addressing is various. It obviously takes into consideration population growth, avoidance of discrimination and the changing route of transmission, but at the same time it also reflects that researchers are not able to clearly understand or arrive at an agreement on whether these people have formed a social organization and how they are organized.

The result is that for years the specific measures of STD prevention have always been swinging or on their own parallel tracks. Those who believe that there are no social organization for people who have high-risk behaviors often emphasize that "Prevention for Everyone, Everybody Counts" (and adolescents in especial), but those who think that the social organization have already been formed would rather aim at those drug addicts and who have multi-partner sex (this in turn focuses on participants in the sex industry and gay sex).

Sadly, the present sociological research work about social stratification and social organization cannot solve problems in the prevention work of AIDS, or even cannot see whether the two guidelines have omissions or biases. "The Theory of Sex Social Network" hasn't appeared until 1994. The theory is that those individuals who have many multiple sexual partner relations are actually networkedly organized by their own interpersonal sexual behaviors. That is to say, though we've never met before and will never meet in the future, me and my sexual partner(s)' sexual partners are objectively existing in a social network of sex which is growing geometrically. If there are someone who have sex relations with both sides of any two social networks of sex, these two networks are connected and form a bigger network. These connectors are called bridge population. Without them, AIDS would not have spread itself to other population. So, they are the key groups of STD prevention work.

The theory of social network of sex actually brings the following three new perspectives to us.

In the first place, the interaction between social factors and individual behavior may not be an equilibrium in the direct and linear reciprocation between society and each individual, nor the interaction between the sea and every drop of water, as is often described. It is more likely that interactions first occur between certain social factors and certain individuals, and then, through the relationships formed between these individuals and others, act successively on other individuals and may eventually diffuse into the entire social network. And vice versa. The behaviors of certain individuals may not affect the society directly and firstly, but can ultimately affect the social factors by continuously acting on other individuals associated with them until it affects a considerable area of the social network.

There is a typical example in AIDS issues: in Western countries, though the propaganda about the use of condoms is seemingly working equally on each individual in society, but only when some individuals from the high-risk population started to use condoms and persuaded their partners to use did the use rate among the whole population increase, and it took almost five years. Then, and only then, will the social repercussions of high-risk population (e.g., oppose panic discrimination) be realized.

Second, in the theory of social network of sex, the perspective of social gender is highlighted. From the statement of the preceding part of the text we can easily find that due to that female have less sexual partners than male, they are more on the fringes of the sexual network than at center, and less likely to become bridge population. That is to say, if AIDS spreads in one of the sexual networks or spread from another network, women will more become passive "end victims". When mother-to-child transmission is taken into account, the harm to women will be doubled.

Looking at "street girls providing sexual service" from this perspective we will find that, though their sexual partners are seemingly a great many and likely to be the chief culprit for spreading AIDS, they are actually on the fringes of the sexual network and less likely to be bridge people, just like other women. That is their real social attribute. Generally speaking, if whoremasters could be faithful to them, the AIDS wouldn't have a chance to spread out of the circle of participants in sex industry.

Such reality can't be simply explained by "men are more promiscuous". It suggests that a male-centered social system is not only reflected in sex, but more likely to be built and developed from sex. In the social network of sex, a man controls sex life of many women, and then namely controls their fertility, and controls the most activities and values of their lives. Finally the whole network will become male-centered when such men increase to a certain extent.

If such networks multiple and get connected, the various social settings that serve it will emerge and become entrenched.

Thirdly, the theory of social network of sex has three colloquial expressions in the perspective of explaining individual behavior: ① Having sex with different people will be in different ways. ② When you have sex with the second person, you are not the original "you". ③ Sex doesn't belong to you or both of you, instead, as soon as you have sex, you two are connected.

There will be no more discussion because though these seem to be pure sexology recognition, they are originally derived from general sociology but use more extreme examples.

In conclusion, the above new perspectives all remind us that, is it possible that the similar condition could exist in other social activities of human? If only because some kind of interaction between many individual behaviors, rather than as a result of the so-called "social decision", these individuals will make up the "network", and in such a "network" to exist in the society and participate in society, so that the "network" with what we used to use class, group between concepts, such as what are the similarities and differences, interaction and structure? Perhaps the social characteristics that we used to value as a class or group of individuals are simply tags that they identify with when they "network" with each other. Once "networking" succeeds, they actually begin to exist and make sense in "networking" units, and the original label (social characteristics) is weakened or changed instead. If so, what kind of people are the "bridge population" between the various "networks"? Why did they succeed in paving the road and building the bridge?

In all, except for "birds of a feather flock together", can people "live in the network"? Or in other words, is social network a tool of one person or a common carrier of many individuals?

In such a society where we rely on friends and network has become the primary capital of getting rich, and the public sphere "nest cases" emerge endlessly, I believe the new perspective brought to us by AIDS is very useful. Perhaps, it can help us to have a deeper understanding of the whole Chinese society.

4.4.2 For the Division Standard and Concept System of Marriage, We Need to Add the Perspective of "Sex"

In the past, even if we didn't study marriage issues purposely, once involved, we still generally and habitually used the most basic classification standards and their conceptual systems in two aspects.

The first aspect is about the classification of marital status. We are accustomed to using a series of categorization that seems to be based on the actual situation of life progress like single, non-marital cohabitated, first married, remarried, multiple married, divorced and widowed. The second aspect is the criteria used to determine the moral nature of sexual relations: marital sexual relations, premarital sexual relations and extramarital sexual relations, or more simplified as sexual relations and non-marital sexual relations.

China's sociology has been using the concept system of "marriage as the basis and morality as the criterion", and seldom studies whether it has enough social authenticity and academic rationality. We often calibrate social phenomena according to concepts, and then investigate and explain them. As a result, many results are consistent with government statistics. It is not only a kind of "blind obedience to the law", but also a kind of "false number calculation", or a kind of "mental suicide". At the same time, because these concepts are often widely used by other people, as a result, many Chinese still believe that the spread of AIDS is "marriage as the boundary".

As for sexual transmission, actually, AIDS is totally "illiterate and legal-illiterate" which do not admit our concept division nor marriage.

It is only related to one fact: have you had sex with a single person or with multiple persons? With a single person you will not be sexually transmitted; if with more than one person, the more the people are, the more likely you are to be sexually transmitted. In other words, even if it is reasonable and legal remarriage, the possibility of sexual transmission is still greater than that of "deviant" but living with a single person unmarried. Similarly, if you are "deviant" but only have extramarital sexual relation with one person, the possibility of sexual transmission is still less than reasonable and legal multiple remarriage.

AIDS also has a potentially long incubation period. Therefore, the question of whether marry with a single person or a number of people is not only a question of "whether you have" in the sense of "marital status" and of present progressive tense, but a question of "whether you have ever had one" in the sense of "marriage history" and of present perfect tense. That is to say, if you have had sex with more than one person, the present divorce and widowhood cannot 100% be the shield against AIDS.

Hence, the sociological recognition of marital issues should add new "sexual" perspective in the era of AIDS.

First, we should establish the basic and core concept of "sexual partner" according to the actual existence of sexual relations (rather than the sociologically legal marriage).

Whether they are in marriage or not, whether their relations are legal or not, as long as they have sex, they are each other's "sexual partner". This is not meant to set up new rules but to exploit new perspectives for us. For example, in view of the phenomenon of "extramarital love" which has long been morally controversial but with little academic research, we believe it will be helpful if we study how society characterize and antagonize "sexual partners" and "spouses" and how the parties internalize or rebel. Furthermore, if these two roles are arranged and combined, maybe we can have a broader and deeper understanding of a series of phenomena from "sex trading" to "keeping mistress", "being close to the rich" to "sexless couple", and explore its social significance, function and operation mechanism.

Further forward, if we fully emphasize the gender factor contained in the concept of "sexual partner", we can get a new understanding by bypassing the embarrassment caused by using the concept of "marriage" when dealing with sexual relations in minority status such as homosexuality.

Then, we should establish a differentiating standard to distinguish relations like "single sexual partnership" and "multiple sexual partnership" instead of the previous "marriage-only demarcation". Thus, we can understand the absurdity of monogamy in social reality and explain the socialization, social operation and historical destiny of the entity existence system of "sex—love—marriage".

4.4.3 Small Social Behaviors of Individuals Should Be Applied to Falsify Theories

According to the theory of rational choice in economics, people will act only when input and output is weighed. Sociology believes that the reasons are much more complicated and broader than this. We have a series of mature theories like cultural script, social structure, social exchange, social interaction and sociodrama. But in the prevention work of AIDS we always meet with some minor questions. For example, when promoting "100% condom use" internationally, there are always some people who do not reach 100%, which can actually be attributed to a variety of small probability, discrete, subtle subjective and objective reasons like the condom package cannot be opened or time is limited, etc. So, does sociology believe these "little things" should be involved in social behaviors? Should and could social theory be applied to analyze these things? Although sociology does not want to and cannot explain 100% of individual's small social behaviors, it can't be an excuse for us not to improve the "interpretation rate".

On the contrary, what is more important is that the AIDS transmission has brought us such a new perspective: though sociology does not necessarily have to be deepened and refined to the level of ethology, all our grand theories should be falsified in individuals' small behaviors, otherwise it may become castles in the air. For example, if someone with a strong sense of preventing diseases doesn't use condom simply because the package cannot be opened, then the theory of cultural script must be supplemented or modified. At least we should add many and even trivial preconditions to the effect of culture on human behaviors. Another example is that no matter what theory we use to explain the behaviors of sexual partners, we must correct it in the process of explaining the "exception" that they do not use condoms just because time is limited instead of immediately turning to another theory to avoid the challenge.

In conclusion, though theory often explains what behavior is, many small social behaviors can explain what theory is not, or at least not applicable to something. That is indeed a good thing for us to develop our theory.

4.4.4 AIDS Gives Us a Push on Empirical Methods

As a matter of common knowledge, the sexual transmission and intravenous drug transmission of AIDS are extremely concealed. Though complete methods are listed in any one of sociological text books, it is still not enough for disease prevention work and requires us to establish specific and operational methods.

For sociology, I am afraid it is still a question of perspective. On the one hand, we often just juxtapose all kinds of methods and combine these methods at most; on the other hand, we often fall into the thinking of the dispute between qualitative research and quantitative research.

Actually, I'm afraid that there are only three methods to empirically understand people's social behaviors. The first is "monitoring", which is the methodological principle adopted by almost every natural science, namely, to find and confirm behaviors through on-scene inspection and measurement. The second method is "confirmation", which is the method adopted by legal circle, that is, using evidence to prove behavior, even if there is no on-scene monitoring. And the last method is "inquiry", which is to determine the behavior according to respondents' complaint which is most commonly used by sociology.

There is no doubt that these three methods are by no means parallel. Whether the collected data is qualitative or quantitative, their authenticity is decreasing. That is to say, even if the best quantitative questionnaire is used, as long as the second method (confirmation) or the third method (inquiry) is adopted, the authenticity of the information obtained is certainly lower than that of the first method (monitoring), even if it is qualitative.

Therefore, as far as the determination of social behavior is concerned, the development direction of empirical research in sociology in China is neither to continue the debate between qualitative and quantitative methods, nor to simply splice various methods in a plane way. Instead, we should try to move from inquiry to confirmation and then to monitoring. Fortunately, the spread of AIDS has forced some researchers to invent new methods, which can be used for reference. For example, the frequency of condom use of both parties involved in the "sex trade" is crucial data in disease prevention work. After years of "inquiring" but still confused, some researchers finally began to purchase used condoms from street girls, and "inquiry" went to "confirmation". For another example, the average daily number of whoremasters received by street girls is also a crucial data. Some researchers first check the chief complaint of street girls with procuress, from "inquiry" to "confirmation" and then observe and record the entry and exit of all whoremasters, and then move to "onitoring".

Of course, it is far from enough to study behavior alone, and most of the non-behavioral phenomena cannot be monitored or even confirmed as the legal circles do. So, please emphasize lie detection with high intensity in "inquiry", because although all lie detection methods cannot make us know what "truth" is, at least it can let us eliminate the false information. In that case, we are on the halfway from "inquiry" to "confirmation".

4.5 The Enlightenment of AIDS Research on Interdisciplinary Perspective

Previously, the author discusses the prevention of AIDS work and sociology between mutual promotion, mutual complement each other in all aspects. Thus, aids sociology also called out.

However, accustomed to reflection of the author, cannot help but be full of doubt: two different disciplines, it is really possible to combine to form a new discipline? What are the conditions for its generation? Thinking all the way down, I wrote this section. It is not about subversion, it is about depth; it is about making us more targeted and more likely to succeed in one fell swoop on the basis of clearer doctrine.

4.5.1 How is Interdiscipline Possible?

Since the 1960s, interdisciplinary as a specialized research object in Europe and the United States has been developed this section focuses on the existing (especially Chinese) literature presented by various types of "interdisciplinary" propositions, does not carry out the analysis of the history of the development of the discipline itself and interrelated. For a discussion of the latter, refer to (US) Wallerstein: Open Social Sciences, Triple Bookstore, 1997, which formed interdiciplinology and was introduced to China in the early 1980s, became an academic hot topic in the 1990s. Its near-terms are transdisciplinary, multidisciplinary, crossdisciplinary, and so on. There are also some references to this meaning, such as subject integration, post-discipline, dedisciplinary and so on. In recent years, interdiscipline in China has been more and more advocated, in various specific fields of application is also increasing, and gradually become an advantage of academic discourse author in the "Chinese Journal Full Text Database" SCI, EL, CSSCI and core journals to "subject" search papers, found from 19 From 90 to the end of 2012, there were 4,216 "interdisciplinary", 7,233 "multidisciplinary", 2,786 "interdisciplinary", 310 "discipline integration" and 31 articles on "going to discipline" or "post-discipline". They come from almost every discipline and research field.

(1) The issue and its new ideas

The author stands on the shoulders of his predecessors to deepen this discussion: How is interdisciplinary possible? On the basis of reflection, we should be alert to the "interdisciplinary proposition" as a trap, and put forward the conditions and prospects for the realization of "interdisciplinary proposition".

The main differences between this section and the existing literature are the following two points.

First of all, this section is not to analyze interdisciplinary research itself, but "interdisciplinary proposition", which is the slogan put forward as the direction of academic development, regardless of the detailed differences within the proposition.

Second, is china's current interdisciplinary research a kind of real (existing), inevitable (coming), or (possible) or just a kind of should (necessary)? Looking at the literature, the results of the interdisciplinary research actually completed are few and far between, and they are not enough to be analyzed and summarized as an objective existence, and most of the literature is based on the assumption of "inevitability" in promoting interdisciplinary and demonstrating its necessity. Although a small number of literatures also discuss interdisciplinary possibilities, they are basically based on the assumption of "possibility". Only one commentator has questioned this hypothesis, but the length is too short to be exhausted.

This section begins with an analysis of why interdisciplinary claims are likely to become a trap, and then explores how they can be made possible.

(2) A brief analysis of the literature

Many literatures are based on two untested assumptions: first, the need for reality or the development of disciplines will inevitably produce interdisciplinary research; They are flawed in logic and have the color of "inevitable". This section is not intended to be discussed.

Interdisciplinary this proposition is Chinese consciously introduced into China, so the author does not try to study its international original ecology, also does not involve differences at home and abroad, but strive to analyze the reality of this proposition in China. Therefore, international literature is not cited for the time being.

(3) Interdisciplinary definition

The general definition in the literature is that interdisciplinary is a new form of research designed to integrate different knowledge into a more comprehensive form of knowledge characterized by strong public perspective orientation and strong problem-solving skills.

Some scholars distinguish between two types of interdisciplinary research. One is the interdisciplinary research carried out within the existing discipline group, that is, the proximity, and the other is the interdisciplinary research between the two major knowledge sectors of natural science and social science, that is, the far edge. Interdisciplinary is often the general term for all interdisciplinary disciplines.

Some literatures are defined by the resulting effects: first, the use of two or more disciplines of mature knowledge to carry out a special problem of interdisciplinary research;

However, there is little disagreement among the large number of papers on the definition of interdisciplinary. So it's not so much a discussion as an introduction.

(4) Interdisciplinary classification

The first type of discussion focuses on "problem-oriented" and summarizes interdisciplinary external and internal conditions. The former mainly refers to the characteristics, compensation, resources and institutional background of the problem to be solved, while the latter mainly refers to the characteristics of the participants, leadership, skills, project organization and intra-group communication.

Another type of discussion emphasizes the importance of "theoretical orientation", pointing out that at the beginning of interdisciplinary cooperation, the theoretical connection between disciplines is the premise, and the design of the subject should take into account the theoretical understanding of different disciplines.

There is also a category of literature that focuses on interdisciplinary studies of immediate neighbours and emphasizes three points. First, it is advocated that all disciplines should recognize the limitations and weaknesses of their own disciplines, so as to establish a "negative equality", that is, "generally weak" sense of equality. Second, in the light of the real society to reflect on the closed weakness of the internal logic of each discipline, in order to establish a "mutual respect and tolerance between the weak" between the various disciplines. Third, as Professor Feng Gang said, the changing nature of the theory must be fully recognized.

(5) Research methods and training, application

In the literature with the theme of "interdisciplinary approach", high-quality papers dealing directly and comprehensively with interdisciplinary research methods are rare.

There are many papers on interdisciplinary construction, management and personnel training. There is also literature devoted to the role of the humanities and social sciences in a particular discipline. But they are actually logical results of the issues discussed in this section, so this section is a little bit more.

(6) A condensed conclusion to the literature

In parallel with great achievements, there are two tendencies in the existing literature: one is pure advocacy and advocacy, and the other is at the technical level. A few papers involve deeper theology, but the depth of analysis is still insufficient.

(7) The practical basis for academic discussion

In recent years, one of the most hot and cutting topics in interdisciplinary studies is the combination of social science and public health, especially in the field of AIDS research and prevention. In China, this combination first came to light around 2000.

The nature of AIDS as a social problem is more prominent than other diseases, coupled with the promotion of international projects and the rise of civil society, so that AIDS can be used as a good example to discuss the combination of social science and public health, so as to extend the analysis and reflection of China's current situation of interdisciplinary issues.

The author's interest in "interdisciplinary" comes more intuitively from his own practice and understanding. Since the 1990s, the author has been actively participating in research and discussion on AIDS at home and abroad as a sociological researcher, and has actually participated in the prevention and treatment of diseases carried out by the public health department, witnessing the interdisciplinary practice in the field of AIDS in China as a direct participant. The author rejoices in his progress, but also deeply feels its limitations, difficulties and challenges.

In order to understand the doubt and explore, the author has been working with the Department of Social Medicine of North Carolina State University in 2007 to explore how to "promote social science research in the field of AIDS in China" and to promote social scientists and public health scholars to carry out specific cooperative research on specific issues with 7 small research projects.

The successful experience is mainly in four aspects: the multidisciplinary world view and methodology began to burst into sparks, the concept of "human" was expanded, the consciousness of "human subjectivity" was promoted, and the possibility of developing data collection methods emerged.

But the main lessons are equally universal. First of all, the research results are basically only one of the problems studied, "cross" into the traditional field of the other side, but the world view and methodology is still the original discipline. Secondly, the result of the implementation path of "cooperation of someone first, cooperation of disciplines" is still basically a list of the results of different disciplines, and the kind of integration and transcendence in the ideal is still unpredictable.

Based on this practice, we have to fundamentally reflect on the idea of interdisciplinary, so this section is available. But due to space constraints, the specific situation is all cut love.

4.5.2 *How Can Interdisciplinary Claims Become Traps?*

(1) Conflicts of worldviews across disciplines

The reason why any relatively mature discipline exists lies first of all in the researchers' high recognition of the world view of the discipline, the formation of "the standardization of disciplines", and the continuous training of beginners, and ultimately the formation of the certainty and passivity of the discipline. This is not only seen as the basis of the entire discipline, but is often implemented as an untested "axiom", although many of its applications are not necessarily clearly aware of this.

The "theoretical link" between the disciplines mentioned in the existing literature has initially touched on this fundamental point, but it is still not clear and in-depth enough. The author thinks that the world view of a discipline is mainly composed of five "meta propositions": the definition of the research object, its identity, its differences, the thinking logic and values in the study.

The meta-proposition of the biomedical discipline group is that it is the world of organisms, and that humans are only one of them. The subjects were "biologically homistic", so the results of animal experiments on any treatment could be applied to humans. The research subjects also have "local differences", so there will be a division of basic medicine, clinical medicine and preventive medicine. In the face of AIDS, biomedical thinking logic tends to "biological problems can only be solved by biological means"; Under the guidance of such five yuan propositions, China's biomedical focus on AIDS treatment and vaccine development, basically not directly involved in prevention work.

China's public health science is basically derived from and affiliated with biomedical science, so its research object is the relatively extensive existence of biological lesions in humans. Its meta-proposition is "the homology of lesions", so there is a "we are prescribing a big prescription" in the subject, that is, the intention to use the same method to deal with a considerable scale of human diseases. In terms of "differences in lesion vectors", it is most inclined to focus on how to determine the possibility of human-to-human behavior of THE spread of AIDS. Its thinking logic tends to "block transmission to prevent", values tend to "prevent disease is the best way to save people", and in practice, it mainly identifies and intervenes in various "high-risk groups".

The early classic "social science" is actually a kind of unremitting efforts to imitate the natural science, but since the 1980s, the world view of "human society research" has been rising day by day. Its meta-proposition regards human beings as the main body of all social phenomena, and its dynamics interact with history and society. It is based first on "the identity of the relationship between man and society" and then on "social differences in the existence of human beings". For AIDS prevention, its thinking logic tends to "solve related social problems in order to better prevent disease", values tend to "human-social coordination is the root of saving people", in practice, it is mainly concerned with those social factors that play a role in disease prevention.

All three university subjects mentioned above study the "human" object, which is necessary for their possible interdisciplinary research. But in terms of adequate conditions, the three universities not only have very different propositions, but also have very different thinking logic and values.

Although "discipline division is a historical mistake … We are the same product of error" (Feng Gang, 2007), but the division of any discipline comes from the rapid development of natural science in recent hundreds of years, its world view is not right or wrong, only differences. In particular, history has proved that discipline division does bring unprecedented human well-being. As a result, the interdisciplinary proposition is on the decline: if the external requirement of any one discipline is born out of shape, then it is not only unrealistic, but also tantamount to denying all existing disciplines.

(2) Bottlenecks in methodology

The differences in research methods in various disciplines not only have differences at the operational level, but also have methodological conflicts.

Biomedical and preventive medicine both follow the basic methodology of general natural science, that is, "objectively determine the truth of the object", but in operation only recognize "the results of repeatable experiments under controlled conditions". Therefore, in the practice of AIDS prevention, public health work can only be based on the existing infection rate to determine who is "high-risk population", but also can only "spread" to the biological definition to take various preventive measures;

Classic social science, since it is impossible to carry out the methodology of natural science mentioned above, can only use various survey methods to learn about the subject's "behavior and its results", and assume it as "objective truth", and then carry out research. But imitation is, after all, mere imitation, and the natural sciences have good reason to think that such research is "unscientific";

The new "human society research" does not try to imitate the natural science, but regards the social phenomenon as the product of the interaction between the subject of "human" and society, history and culture. Therefore, its research data is not only "the result of the survey", but "the construction of the human subject", especially the meaning of people's own "behavior and its results" made calibration. In the methodology of natural science, this is simply the opposite, and the necessary conditions for interdisciplinary research have been lost.

In this regard, the current literature mainly advocates three directions of effort: overcoming the "interdisciplinary paradox"; But the discussion of "how possible" has not gone far enough to move progress forward.

(3) The origin of the trap

The above analysis is not to deny the interdisciplinary proposition, but to try to start from the "impossible" hypothesis, to demonstrate that the proposition is likely not to understand their own target exactly—many researchers do not actually understand and understand the various disciplines of the world view and methodology, not to recognize the differences and their meaning, just stay in the "good things should be done" cognitive level, and even show "call more natural people will do" tendency.

This is likely to become a trap.

At the operational level, if researchers simply because "useful" on the rush to invest in some kind of interdisciplinary research, for the various disciplines involved in the world view but lack of a profound understanding, then it can only be futile, and may even be in order to get "output" and pieced together, to create a "building blocks" type of simple list, do not have intrinsic connections and behavior logic, or even pull the flag to do tiger skin results, in people are harmful.

Thus, at the level of cooperation, there will be a "strong discipline eats the weak subject" practice or worry about it. In particular, if interdisciplinary claims are still tied to adjusting academic relationships, or even just interpersonal relationships, then the best outcome is just a bed-and-bed dream in an arranged marriage.

At the theoretical level, if the above-mentioned mistakes become the norm or even mainstream, then its output will not only be difficult to become academic achievements, but also self-binding, blocking the progress of various disciplines.

At the level of social effects, blind interdisciplinary proposition, if it really becomes an academic or even social discourse, then it will take considerable power to influence or even dominate the existing research lines of various disciplines, which is likely to cause unpredictable damage. In particular, if this trend of thought unfortunately becomes a market demand or even administrative demand, it may induce more researchers to blindly invest in it, and may even distort the overall direction of academic development. In the impetuous current China, this is by no means a worry.

(4) Existing policy propositions are difficult to leap out of the trap

The discussion above is really about "what is called interdisciplinary", but the problem goes far beyond that.

① What kind of subjects do you cross?

Interdisciplinary propositions tend to be based on the division of existing disciplines. Its meta-proposition is: the existing division of disciplines is still possible, but the need to "cross" it. However, in China's reality, there is a set of first-level disciplines, second-level disciplines, branch disciplines, research direction of such a set of quite administrative concept system and operating mechanism. At what level do we advocate "crossing"? Even, does this need us to advocate? For example, there is no first-level discipline of psychology in the National Standard Discipline Code. Thirty-six secondary disciplines with the word psychology are subserrated into 18 different primary disciplines, while the second-level disciplines indicating sociology are distributed among eight primary disciplines and physiology is dispersed among the five first-level disciplines. According to such regulations, psychology and sociology are inherently interdisciplinary, and cross the most basic classification of the first-level disciplines.

Of course, the author believes that the interdisciplinary proposition mainly refers to the subject that should be divided according to the thexiom. But in real life, many researchers publish articles or evaluation of job titles, often by the above-mentioned disciplines of the division of the thymis or even damage. Therefore, while advocating purely academic interdisciplinaryism may promote the improvement of national discipline division, that is another problem that does not contribute to the realization of its ideas.

② Who and who "cross"?

Interdisciplinary propositions are basically based on the similarity of the subjects. This can easily be understood as the possibility or even inevitability of being interdisciplinary as long as both disciplines are studying the same problem. The assumption is that the same research can be done on the same subject, but it is divided into existing disciplines.

But two questions ensue: first, can this hypothesis be tested? Second, which subject is still unified?

In terms of sociology alone, the debate of some different schools has already reached the level of world view and methodology, showing the situation of "different ways, no common seeking" or even "not wearing days together". This is also the case in other disciplines. So, should sociology be "cross" with another subject, or should sociology's own schools "cross"? Or simply two scholars "cross"? In the absence of discussion, interdisciplinary slogans are inevitably hollow.

③ How can the same person "cross"?

The best answer to these questions is that all-round, interdisciplinary talent should be developed from the start. This is well-intentioned, but logically it is this: if you learn any subject well must follow the world view and methodology of that discipline, then learning both disciplines at the same time cannot naturally achieve interdisciplinary, but the opposite. So this person must break the premise of the above logic and be a traitor in both disciplines.

So the real question should actually be: can any discipline tolerate or even encourage "non-business" and "non-conformity with academic norms" of future generations?

4.5.3 Three Levels of Conditions to Realize Interdiscipline

(1) Necessary conditions

First of all, we need to clarify a historical fact: the existing research direction or research results with interdisciplinary possibilities are often not the result of the intentional actions of people in different disciplines, let alone the invasion or transformation of other disciplines;

The most typical example is: in the long process of the medical model from a purely biological model to a biological psychosocial model, not only without the participation of any other discipline, even the greater impact cannot be talked about. Because in the historical situation of discipline isolation, neither side will pay attention to what the other is saying, let alone allow the other side to "step in".

The shift in medical models stems from the mainstreaming of heresy within the medical community. Engel, an American professor of psychiatry, first raised the issue of "big reversal" in 1977. At the time, the mainstream of psychiatry as a whole was an attempt to return to biomedical science, which had a clearly defined academic basis for reduction theory and strongly attracted psychiatry, which had been considered "unscientific". Engel in order to oppose this tendency, simply the biomedical overall subversion, but did not expect to be deafening, quickly mainstreamed, to the medical profession brought spring.

This history tells us that interdisciplinary needs conditions.

Necessary: "Heresy thought" can survive within the discipline.

Full condition: There must be a number of "heresy molecules" as carriers, they must be self-indulgent edge, enjoy it.

Conditions for development: "heresy" must be mainstreamed.

Thus, the subject itself has a qualitative change, will appear to absorb other disciplines of the world view and methodology of the possibility.

However, this still does not necessarily lead to interdisciplinary appeals.

"Heresy" initially simply adheres to "heresy", often with no other choice, and can only develop into interdisciplinary action if it discovers that its heresy is in common with another discipline. In particular, the probability of this happening is not very large, many "heretics", their lives are still in the discipline of hard work, and did not attempt to spy on other disciplines. This means that the sufficient condition for interdisciplinary basis is that the "heresy" within any discipline must also be open to discipline.

If so, when any two disciplines produce the need for cross-integration, it is difficult to produce between the "big pressure small" or "university hegemony". It's not that it shouldn't be, it's that it's impossible Because both sides are "heresy" origin, both have the openness of the subject, it does not matter the size. If the opposite happens, the most fundamental reason is that the bullying party is not really a heresy, or does not have a real heresy. At present, in China's AIDS prevention practice, interdisciplinary research is not satisfactory, also does not come from this.

In the final analysis, the reason why interdisciplinary research is possible is not only from the opening up of each discipline, but from the diversity and equality of its own disciplines. What we need is not only to eliminate the isolation between disciplines, but also to demand the right to free development within disciplines. Interdisciplinary research is really open heresy in the breakout unexpectedly meet and love at first sight.

In this case, interdisciplinary claims have the potential to raise pseudo-questions. The real problem is that each family is allowed to tear down its own walls, allow "elopement" and "wild marriage", rather than preaching to challenge other people's boundaries.

Scholars often say: any subject, research to the end is philosophy. This suggests that people have actually been assuming that all disciplines may actually have a "meta" point that is sufficiently connected, but we rarely explore such a meta-problem and do not realize that it is not only an interdisciplinary theoretical fulcrum, but also a starting point for research.

(2) Adequate conditions

In the process of creating interdisciplinary research, the heretics of each discipline actually have their inherent behavior logic, which is to create at least three aspects of the new meta-proposition. The following is illustrated by the presentation in the field of AIDS prevention.

First, create a world view that is different from the original discipline.

In the meta-proposition of the subject and its hombiality and difference, biomedical science must accept human "social differences" (different populations are not the same likely to be infected) while adhering to "biological hom identity" (the AIDS-positive test is applicable to anyone). On the contrary, no matter how much emphasis is placed on the great role of society and culture, the study of human society will not deny the epidemic situation of AIDS. Therefore, the two sides will be "high-risk groups" on the basis of the effective concept of a new meta-proposition: disease and its spread does not originate but exists in society. This avoids both "social factor unrelated theory" and "biological factor cancellation theory", which has at least begun to constitute a platform for dialogue among various disciplines.

In the work practice, it is precisely because of such a new meta-proposition, so public health personnel will go deep into a variety of high-risk groups, understand and understand their knowledge, attitudes, beliefs and behavior, not just "see a doctor and cure." Similarly, human society researchers are based on the new meta-proposition, began to actively participate in the treatment of people living with HIV practice, rather than "not in their place, do not seek their own politics."

Second, in the logic of thinking, the two sides have also found a meta-proposition with commonalities: physiological conditions and behavioral characteristics are constructed from each other. It is precisely because both sides accept this proposition, public health personnel will strive to explore the infection and high-risk groups of medical behavior, and humanities and social researchers will continue to advocate the prevention and treatment of gynaecological diseases into the "Miss" AIDS prevention work.

Third, at the level of value orientation, the two sides have gone beyond the "care for life" this original common ground, deep into the new meta-proposition: life lies in existence, but also in quality. As a result, many public health personnel have "crossed the line" to help infected people solve the problem of health insurance or low insurance, while human society researchers have delved into the situation of drug use of infected people.

Thus, the author can think that in the field of AIDS prevention, a new discipline combining public health and humanities and social research is being formed. Although it is only sprayed out, but its direction is no longer in doubt.

(3) Conditions for development: new methodologies

Historically, the emergence of almost every discipline in the natural sciences has been based on the success of a new research method. Therefore, interdisciplinary research needs to explore a common methodology, which is its development conditions. Example: Someone has been biomedically diagnosed with AIDS, but psychologically he has no feelings and does not agree with himself, and lives in a social environment without any pressure on AIDS. So he's not an infected person? If judged only by the worldview of three established disciplines, it must not only be a mess, but no one can answer: is this state of certainty? Is this an expression of "holistic"? Is this a "new knowledge"?

Further from the methodological level, the medical test for this person is "objective determination", his feelings and approval is based on his "main complaint", the description of his social environment is derived from other people's social. So, are the results of these three different research methods comparable, categoristic and inductive? In the final analysis, the methodology of objective determination and the methodology of summary, since separation and even isolation, and thus brought unprecedented human welfare, then we now have a good reason to ask these two methodologies to "cross"? How can we feel if the result of the "cross" is more likely to be defeated?

In order to solve this logical dilemma, we have to discuss the problem from the basis of epistemology. The author is not talented, at present can only ask the following questions to teach the reader.

First, the relentless pursuit of certainty is the objective law of human cognition, or is it the overlord clause produced by certain disciplines for self-incrimination and self-preservation? Or is it the cult instilled in discipline hegemony? Why can't the object of academic research be "foggy existence" (dispersed, dynamic, perceived by the subject)?

Second, for human beings, what we "objectively measure" is really the objective world, or is it because we ignore the difference between "the other world" and "my world"?

Thirdly, is there anything that our subjects are not classified, that they should not be classified, that they should not be classified? Why do we lack a minimum sensitivity to "unclassified status"?

Of course, the author firmly opposes agnosticism. The crux of the problem lies in the lack of cognitive tools and expressions for any kind of "non-objective determination", not only the lack of conceptual system, but also the lack of logic of argumentation, but also lack of comparison and definition with objective measurement methodology. Therefore, despite the efforts of researchers in various disciplines, this lack still comes mainly from the unfinished power, cannot blame the "discourse hegemony".

(4) The conclusion

The author thinks that there are "heresy" in the original discipline, interdisciplinary research has the possibility to produce, all aspects of "heresy" break out and converge into a river, interdisciplinary research can be achieved, and the participants take the initiative to challenge the methodology of the original discipline, interdisciplinary research can continue to develop.

4.5.4 What is the Feasibility of Interdiscipline?

(1) Promoting "meta-research"

Researchers in all disciplines need to first have a thorough understanding of what the philosophy of their subject is.

In the history of the world, this "meta-study" is often carried out by experts in the history of disciplines, which has produced a series of brilliant achievements, and is a long way ahead of the natural sciences. However, in the current Chinese academic circles, enough to sum up their own disciplines of world view and methodology scholars are still not enough, they create knowledge, even in this discipline is still not popular enough.

In particular, many philosophical generalizations of this discipline, still based on the idea of discipline division, tend to focus on their own connotation and extension, independence, their own social values, and so on, but often lack of their own and other disciplines of commonalities. In China's discipline division system, this has the understandable necessity of "survival and development", but objectively it is inevitable to form a strict barrier to interdisciplinary research.

The author's ideal state is: in the student stage, it is enough to recognize the philosophy of the subject, and at least the same degree of recognition of the philosophy of at least one other subject. It would be best if you could get to know your heart and blurt it out.

(2) Seek commonalities

The world view and methodology of the disciplines within the discipline group may have more in common. But this is not inevitable, nor is it the nor nor is it the nor nor is it normal, neither falling from the sky nor because of "arranged marriage" and beauty. The most typical example is that Western medicine and Traditional Chinese medicine, no matter how similar they are in subject affiliation, are still distinguished or even tit-for-tat because of differences in fundamental philosophy.

In particular, it is worth thinking about: at a time when interdisciplinary propositions are on the rise, the boom in the creation of new disciplines or new differentiation of disciplines is also booming, with 1,979 "subjects" searched for academic papers on "themes" in almost all fields of research, and 1,979 "subject differentiations" found. So is there something in common between the two? This requires exploring and not having a successful guarantee. This makes it the second step in interdisciplinary research.

(3) Full presentation of the mandatory provisions

First, "light up the weakness", showing the weakness of the subject. This is because existing disciplines can be established largely on the provision of more research that is logical enough, while a variety of failures, abandonments, omissions, fallacies and losses are often kept secret or left behind as "academic privacy". Interdisciplinary research is about doing the opposite, forcing every discipline to reflect by "fully presenting" the new rigid rule. Thus, any cross-cutting, penetration and fusion is sufficient.

Second, "analysing others" means that we must not only list the different research results of different disciplines on a problem, but must introduce and analyze the world view of other disciplines. It is best to be able to find the differences and the results of the differences.

Third, "presenting methodology" is not only the need to reflect on the methodology of the original discipline, but also must be able to find even a little desirability from other disciplines, and to large books. For example, in the study to investigate the AIDS epidemic, public health personnel in the use of questionnaires, has begun to affirm and seek qualitative interview methods, in order to learn the differences and richness of the subjects of the survey, greatly promoting the progress of research and specific work. This suggests that interdisciplinary first and forth is to allow the exploration of new methodologies to begin. From this point of view, the difference between the interdisciplinary theoretical orientation and problem orientation, which is of general concern to the existing literature, has not only lost the significance of the discussion, but also the basis of classification. Only the orientation of methodology is the only real problem that can be better solved by using interdisciplinary research.

The value of full presentation lies in the fact that interdisciplinary research is first and forequist providing such a context for discussion and a new way of thinking. This is not only a new starting point, but also a new knowledge in itself. It affects not only researchers, but readers, and thus their successors.

In particular, this complete presentation should become a rigid academic norm. In this way, the results presented completely are no longer what a single discipline can do, nor belong to any of the original disciplines, but an equal dialogue between disciplines.

(4) The only criterion for evaluation: reflection on the original discipline

If we agree that the nature of interdisciplinary research is to produce new knowledge in a "second way", then it should not be from the end of the "Yangtze River after the waves forward", but should be a different way of "willow dark flowers and a village", or inclusive "sea moon tide", preferably the "Yellow River water coming out of the sky."

The author's proposition is obvious, without reflection on the original discipline, there is no interdisciplinary existence. In particular, such reflection, while not necessarily leading to interdisciplinary results, is bound to promote openness, diversity and sustainable development in all disciplines.

(5) Interdisciplinary inappropriately as the goal of subjective efforts

Reflection on this discipline presents four possibilities, and never just one. The first possibility is that if the commonalities between the original discipline and other disciplines can be sought, it will become interdisciplinary research. The second possibility is that if it is not possible, the researchers will have to find a different way to create a new discipline. The third possibility is that the questioning of the discipline merely promotes its development, but does not achieve interdisciplinarity and does not create new disciplines. The fourth possibility is to contribute to the death of the subject, just as everything is like street fortune-telling.

For the foreseeable future, we don't have any evidence to determine which possibility is more likely to occur. Therefore, from the construction process, the existing interdisciplinary practice is actually more of an unexpected result, rather than the original goal of self-conscious struggle.

If "interdisciplinary" is the goal of subjective efforts in the first place, then objectively it is tantamount to advocating only the first possibility of academic development, but also involuntarily suppressing the other three development possibilities. The result: this new proposition is actually very likely to undermine academic diversity and diversity, or interfere with the development of the original discipline.

It is not an operational question, but a new level of awareness, to promote the four development possibilities of various disciplines in an all-round way, rather than simply advocating interdisciplinary approaches with quick success. It directs participants to strip away all appearances (such as the social needs, power relations, organizational management, etc.) and points directly to the core of the problem: differences and coordination between worldviews and methodologies. This can greatly enhance participants' predictability of interdisciplinary possibilities and avoid the "failure before the beginning" tragedy.

In summary, the interdisciplinary value goal should be: to provide a holistic situation of equal competition for the "heresy" in each discipline, not to construct the interdisciplinary goal into an exclusive religious belief, let alone to build a unified world of dissolving pluralism again under the banner of integration.

For the subject discussed in this book, the creation of "AIDS sociology", first of all, soberly and deeply recognized and frankly acknowledge the conflict between the two disciplines of meta-propositions, meta-assumptions and meta-philosophy, before it is possible to jointly build our new discipline. In this regard, the author has some thinking, but still contains a lot to put, so put it into the "Postscript" inside to say it.

Postscript

The social construction of AIDS in the sociology of life has traditionally been a part of preventive medicine and public health. But from the perspective of creating "AIDS sociology", it is actually one of the components of the whole health cause. Its ultimate goal is to make its due contribution to the overall health of all people. At present, China has appeared the "health sociology" reference, many scholars are working hard to promote the development of this new discipline. Therefore, the social science of AIDS into the scope of health sociology, it seems beautiful.

But this leads to a basic academic question: What exactly is health? If we do not understand this problem, then the development direction of AIDS sociology will be confused, unsustainable, and may even take the sword away.

There are two distinct international arguments for the definition of health.

One is traditional scholars who insist that so-called health must be determined from a biological and medical perspective, using biological and medical means, and based on biological and medical test results. Even China's recently burse concept of "sub-health" is strictly following the above definition.

Another group of scholars argues that health is not a health, but a well-being, "good". The World Health Organization defined it in 1998 as: "Health is not only disease-free or infirm, but also a state of physical and mental happiness and social well-being".

Around 2000, this group of scholars once again put forward the concept of "health from the perspective of individual rights", including the following: "Good" is not a medical can be objectively measured things. It is a personal value that cannot be measured by any uniform "value neutrality" standard. The right of individuals to recreation is a prerequisite for health.

In English, well-being refers to a good state, a good feeling, is a high-level abstract word, very common in the English world. But it lacks the most appropriate counterpart in the Chinese, which can be translated as "well-being" or "happiness" or even "welfare". The reason why I translate as "good" is to avoid the word "kang", in order to highlight the "good" such a state. In fact, the translation of "euthanasia" may be

S. Pan, *The Social Construction of AIDS Issues*, A Sociological View of AIDS,
https://doi.org/10.1007/978-981-16-7519-5

better, but because the word "euthanasia" is already very popular in China, so we have to avoid it.

Replacing "health" with the concept of "good" is of great academic and historical significance.

First of all, health refers only to physical good condition, goodness includes the happiness of the mind. Especially in Chinese, safety, tranquility, well-being of these words, "An" is very important, all expressed in the physiological health outside of a subjective feeling and life experience of "good".

Second, there is no inevitable causal relationship between well-being and health, not the question of who produces or decides who, but the good state that human beings need at the same time. In layman's terms, people with physical health may not have a good life;

Third, health is medicine to evaluate you, and well-being is your own experience, feelings, evaluation and recognition.

This raises a question of on-the-body philosophical significance: Who should judge my own state of existence? Apart from medicine (including science in a broad sense), why does my human body's feelings count? If there is a contradiction or even a conflict between the two assessments, then how on earth am I?

In Chinese, the expression "feels good" has been used as a negative and sarcastic term, a manifestation of subjective idealism, regardless of objective facts. But that's right, isn't it? Should it be the same? In particular, in the "subject construction perspective" Pan Yuming, Huang Yingying: "subject construction": the revolution and local development space of the perspective of sexual sociology research, Sociological Research, No. 3 of 2007. It seems that this is precisely the chinese society's long-standing myth.

Let me give an example of my most professional "sex study", which cites statistical charts from the results of four national random sample surveys I have conducted (see Fig. 3.1 and Fig. 3.8).

The question I ask is that the following statistics that Chinese encounter in their sex lives are designed to illustrate the difference between "healthy" and "well-being" and therefore do not analyze or discuss the specific problems they reflect. Are they all physiological lesions or disorders? Are they all medically determined to be "unhealthy"? However, they do weaken the "good" and "sexual well-off" of Chinese.

Figure 3.1: Sexual fantasy in sex in addition to Fig. 3.2 pretend to reach orgasm. Figure 3.3: Very few daily intimate. Figure 3.4: never caress. Figure 3.5: sex life shame. Figure 3.6: feel that sex dirty. Figure 3.7: himself was reluctantly sex life. Figure 3.8: never communicate sex life experience similar to many other situations, such as women lack of orgasm, sex monotony poor, do not understand the emotional communication in caressing, do not know respect for each other's wishes, unwilling to work hard for each other's sexual pleasure ... No physiology book has judged them "unhealthy" and no traditional doctor has "treated" them. But people in their daily lives no doubt regard these situations as "bad"

Therefore, the conclusion is obvious: health is only a medical judgment, "good" is the determination of the society in which we live. The two are indispensable, cannot be negated or replaced by each other.

But why does the concept of health become a one-man or even a discourse hegemony? Has it actually become the last ideological weapon of social discipline? This requires reflection: who is judging whose sexual health is being determined? Why must such a person judge others? What is the value objective of the decider? Why did you get this far? These are on-subject discussions, and this book is no longer on the way.

Back to the issue of AIDS, then the creation of AIDS sociology, should health as their academic basis, or should be good as their goal?

This is of great practical significance in the first place. For a long time, in the specific work of aids, AIDS-infected people have been relatively absent. Their world, their lives, their hearts, have not received enough attention and research. What they ask for, what we can help them achieve, is healthy or well? Even if the current drugs can suppress the onset of AIDS, but they can expect to be healthy again? Can we help them get healthy? In real life, what they need more is to be well and to reduce the discrimination, difficulties and troubles that come with being infected. That's what we're most likely to do and do well.

Secondly, from a scientific point of view, no matter how hard AIDS sociology and preventive medicine combined, it is based on sociology, can not solve the medical definition of health problems. However, it is more likely to promote well-off under the social definition. In this regard, we have enough historical success.

In the 1970s, the Boston Women's Health Writing Collective, an American women's non-governmental organization, independently constructed women's own perceptions of physical, disease, and health concepts, and wrote the book "Our Bodies, Ourselves", which promoted the well-being of generations of American women.

This is a more life-like and universal collective writing experience, including taking care of ourselves, intimacy and sex, fertility three major content. It involves women's body image, mood, psychology, and other issues, including women's accounts of sexual relationships, and encouraging us to speak out about our physical condition and experiences with doctors: how to have children, how to use contraception, how to have abortions. It records many women's experiences of self-care, treatment and nursing, and tells many stories of women's deep understanding of life and body.

The book was written collectively, expanding from more than 30 women to more than 500 in Boston and eventually to thousands of women, creating the "Our Body, Ourselves" women's health movement in the United States. The book has been welcomed and valued by women in various countries and is regarded as "the most important work born in the women's movement". Its characteristics and writing style can also be illustrated by an introduction to the book:

"...The reader seems to be at a crowded and comfortable table, holding a cup of coffee in hand, and joining a heated discussion: this is the doctor's opinion, this is the midwife's consideration, this is an ordinary woman's own experience. Gradually, the reader seems to hear his voice and joins the discussion: in my case. As an equal, that is, to regard their own experience as a kind of knowledge for others to learn from, this is not only a process of education, but also a process of self-empowerment."

Not only has the book been revised in the United States for at least 6 editions, published for more than 30 years, made into Braille, audio-visual version, into the "health gate" of the computer data network, and has been translated or adapted into at least 15 languages, distributed more than 4 million copies worldwide, far-reaching worldwide. The book was first introduced to China by Chinese feminists in the 1980s and was published in 1989 as an official translation of Chinese.

Learn from such successful experience, AIDS sociology should also be able to mobilize AIDS patients to write their own such a book, present their own lives, exchange their feelings and experiences, refine their own efforts to strive for good experience and lessons, spread their own "to die" concept of life. In this way, not only other infected people can benefit and cheer up, but also to the whole society to preach the value and significance of life, improve the current prevalence of China's "fear of death but do not understand death, will die but not good at death" bad situation.

At this point, the main thrust of my "Travel" is also logical: the sociological research needs to fight AIDS and can gradually move towards AIDS sociology, AIDS sociology should and may one day reach the "sociology of life" higher realm.

I dare to guess: the sociology of life is to put human life in the historical process and specific circumstances, to include as many social factors as possible, to sociologically unique research methods, to analyze the biological mechanism of life this necessary condition, in what kind of social practice this control condition, through which human subject construction and active choice to become a sufficient condition, and ultimately form the existing value and significance, and then in what kind of information and feedback under this development condition, constantly dynamic changes.

If so, this life is enough.

Appendix
Fieldwork and Insights into Sexual Transmission

The following nouns, such as "underground sex industry", "red-light district" (an area driven by prostitution), "street girl", "whoremaster", "procuress" and "pimp", have to be used only for the sake of academic research and the real situation. They are not formal terms, nor do they represent the values of the author and publisher.

(1) I am on site: "experiences of getting along with street girls"

At first, I was just like an "escort boy" and accompanied "capitalists" to run around. In 1995 or so, a friend of mine became a nouveau riche. After being rich, he took me to enjoy beer and skittles, regarding me as a "trophy man". We knew each other during the "Cultural Revolution" when we worked in the same factory. After making a small fortune, he took me to travel more than a dozen places in both south and north of China. Accidentally, I came into contact with some street girls. But after that, I just notice them in many places. Everyone has the curiosity and would like to know something about them. So do I. Therefore, I tried to talk with them face to face, only to find that it didn't work. It seemed as if there was a high mountain between us. I got nothing.

I kept racking my brain for ways to get things done. Then I realized it entailed a boss and a procuress. Only in that way could I get in touch with some street girls. However, where were they? How could I find them? In 1998, my childhood friend became the president of a hospital in Dongguan, Guangdong. Being a president, he knew a lot of people. In addition, many of his patients were doing business who boasted the wide network of people as well. He knew well the boss and procuress of a Karaoke lounge and offered to introduce me to them. That was how I began my research. Academically, we call him the GUIDE.

However, I had no access to other places but the Karaoke lounge itself. So, that was the only place where I could meet street girls and got on with them. As a friend of the boss and procuress, I went there every day and the street girls knew I was not a whoremaster. I lodged there for a total of 47 days. It was really a long time but that was the only way to know something. Because people only show their authentic selves in non-working hours, occasions and relationships.

S. Pan, *The Social Construction of AIDS Issues*, A Sociological View of AIDS,
https://doi.org/10.1007/978-981-16-7519-5

Before I went to the Karaoke lounge, I had already understood that it made no sense to pretend as a whoremaster. Pretending as a whoremaster was totally wrong from the root and through that I could only know the price range at best. But did I need to make efforts to know that? Everybody knew it, ok? If I had pretended to go whoring, I would have seen the professional performances like models and movie actors. That was not the real side of them.

I would like to know something about street girls. At first, I intended to figure out the reason why they took such a post, which many people wanted to know, because they seemed just like other common people. A year later, I found that was really a stupid question. It was just like asking a soldier the reason why they went to the frontline in a war—"Cuz I love my motherland"—that had no point at all. However, I only realized it after getting along with those street girls.

"Why do you study this? I can't understand."—street girls wouldn't ask such questions like scholars. The first they wanted to know was "Are you an undercover or a policeman?" For that, the boss and procuress could testify I was not. The second was "Are you a reporter?". The reporters were their second most hatred, and if the reporters came, street girl would almost strangle them to death. Then I told them the reason why I came there. They had never thought it was a research and they even didn't know "research" this word. When the boss introduced me to others, he said: "First, he's from Beijing; second, he's a professor now and will soon become a 'researcher'." I came back and told that to my colleagues and they all laughed. For people in that community, they knew relatively more about "professors" than about "researcher", so researchers were superior to professors.

"What are you going to do here?" That question had its answer on the third day, and street girls explained it with their own understanding. I said: "I just come to have a look." They got it and said, "You just look but don't have sex". Then they comprehended that and accepted me.

In fact, for most people from the bottom, their life is very simple, and the world is extremely small. Street girls judged a person by whether he or she might harm them as police and reporters did, but I was just a "passenger". They didn't care whether I was a psychopath or had any addictions because they had no awareness of those.

The first procuress graduated from high school and later received some correspondence courses. She was worried that I would put her in my book. But none of her street girls had thought of that, and they all said, "Oh, it's so great. Write me in your book and use my real name". Then they told me their names, but I soon forgot. (Not just for keeping their privacy, but for not remembering their names. That is our basic ethical principle in a research.)

They really wanted to be in a book. Because they seldom received any attention, even from their parents, they were so happy after knowing they might be in my book. But some elder street girls, half of them having children, might have some scruples, for they were afraid that would make trouble to their kids. The less-educated didn't understand what it meant to be written in a book and made no comments about that.

How did I deal with such worry? It was too simple. I came back there a year later and gave her my book. She was so happy and looked through for a long time. "Ah, I can't tell that is me." Then she transferred it to the Taiwan boss.

After a few days, I realized their lives were too restricted. Street girls were experiencing oppression, exploitation and sexual assaults. Besides that, their life was extremely boring. They were tired of watching TV but didn't have enough money to play mahjong even it was only 1 yuan for one round. So, there was no mahjong, no poker. They had nothing to do but sitting there waiting for guests who might come at any time, deadly bored. Doing that for a long time, the street girls became highly sluggish. They hoped to have someone to talk with, but not a whoremaster, because they have to "perform" in front of their guests. The younger street girls are, the more they were desirous of having someone to chat with. Many middle-aged street girls had children and carried heavy psychological burden for they couldn't rear their kids under such atmosphere. To build our relationship, I chatted and played cards with them and made fortune-telling through palm-reading for them.

From 1998 to 2010. I went to 13 such kind of "Karaoke lounge" in total, and came into contact with more than 1,000 street girls. Though I couldn't recall all in detail, I still remember the general context. For example, if I took out a story about street girl in my book, I could remember where she roughly came from, or at least where she was at that time.

Only for the first two s I went there alone, and then I went with my students. I took 7 girls at most and 4 at least. What is the merit of taking girls? They could talk about emotional problems together. Why was it also easy for me to talk with them? Because there was a generation gap and age gap between me and street girls. When I had lived in karaoke lounge for two days, the street girls got to know me and they even called me daddy or grandpa because I looked too old. The age gap gave them security and that was very useful. They didn't take me as a whoremaster-though there were indeed some older whoremasters and treated me as their elders. They even offered to tell me about their own stories.

I keep saying that treating street girl as common people, but at the beginning I wasn't conscious of that. I have written a total of six books on street girls and figured that out in the third or fourth book.

(2) The roots of sexual transmission

Though "Red-light districts" are illegal yet it has its definition. The first is geographically concentrated, the second is relatively open. And for the third, it should be a pure prostitution platform without any other sundry stuff. "Districts" meeting standards above are not that much, but they, no matter big or small, emerge in each town. If there are three such kind of "Karaoke lounge", it can be called "red light districts". Three lounges form a small "red-light district", 30 forms a big one, but 300 is impossible or it would be too lawless.

That was true at least in Sichuan. We explored development zones in 11 counties there, all of which had "red light districts". The world largest agricultural county there only had an industrial item, a paper mill. The government would like to establish a development zone in that country but only invested to build a road. The rest relied on farmers and citizens. They were called on to build houses using their own money in the development zone.

I, even as the layman of economics, knew that no one would invest in that country which had an hour's drive from Chengdu (the capital of Sichuan). Without materials and the technology, only the lunatics could invest there. That country was densely populated with tens of thousands of people. After the development zone was established, all people began to set up stalls, leaving no hand for farming. Three months later, they discovered there were more people selling than buying. Eventually, the farmer had no methods but established "red-light district", because only street girls could attract people to come over.

At the beginning, the local government banned the district's operations. Later, tax officials realized they owed a great debt to farmers. And the mayor frankly said that street girls drove one-third of the economy. Because of them, the government could get taxes, farmers could live, and food and clothes business could thrive. In my book Why Red-Light Districts Exist in China, I showed that it was because of this GDP-ism which drove the government blindly built development zones.

Later I found the boss did an excellent job in ideological work. How did they guide street girls? They said to them: "Look at all these men coming in and out, seeming like a good and decent man? When they come home, they are all best husbands, and when they meet their children, they are all excellent fathers. What is your future prospect? Living with such kind of men? But they even don't want to marry you! Your highest ambition is no more than to marry a city dweller and good husband who will be a good father when you have kids, right? If he comes here for you, what could you do? Their wives don't know what their husbands have done here and no one else does. Even they know, they still pretend they have no idea, but you know that and see it every day."

Then street girls' conviction would be shattered completely. For low-educated street girls, they are unable to express in that way, but her only faith is indeed love and marriage. The lower bottom the street girls are from, the less money, connections and opportunities they have, and the more likely she is to believe love and marriage. If you tell them the marriage is unreliable, she will do anything without being taught or forced.

Besides that, the boss had another trick. "Do you want to run away? Ok. How much money do you have? 30 yuan? How far can you go with that? You even cannot afford the ticket! Without money to buy food, you have to come back to seek help. And if you end up getting home, I will call your village head! By that time, your whole family will be suffered humiliation. You may want to charge me now. Ok, go out and turn left to the police station, and tell them your job at first!" Having no way to go, they have to do sexual affairs without coercion which is against their stereotype. I saw and heard all those with my own eyes and ears.

In Sichuan, the procuress and bosses went to the labour market in Chengdu to recruit "girls". Nominally, they wanted to employ some waitresses and told them they would work in a small karaoke lounge and all they needed to do was just playing discs and serving the dishes. The young girl knew nothing about the inside story but expected to be hired. On the way to work, the boss would chat with the girl to figure out whether she was a street girl before. If she was, the thing would become simple, but if not, he would treat her to dinner and bought her some beautiful clothes, saying the place she would to work was an upscale place. Though the little girl knew nothing behind the scenes, she accepted the job. She would serve dishes the first day, and then was brainwashed: "Look at the girls around you, look at their food and clothes and earnings. What about you? You just make 100 yuan a month. Why? Because we cover your food and accommodation which cost a lot. So, you just have 100 yuan a month. Do you accept that?".

"100 yuan a month? I would rather die than do it", the girl might say. The boss would reply: "Ok, just go away but remember to return my money for your food and clothes. The food costs 20 yuan and the clothes cost 100 yuan, and all together is 120 yuan. You know, it is worth that money. Give me 120 yuan and you can go home". The boss believed there was no more than 50 yuan in girl's pocket, so she could not afford 120 yuan. "If you could not afford that, you need to serve dishes to pay back my money. But I will only give you 100 yuan a month with free food and accommodation." Within five days, she would offer to do sex service. Then the boss would tell her: "I know you're a virgin. The first time values 5,000 yuan. Other girls earn 2, 000 yuan a month, but you can make more than twice money at one time." I didn't know such kind of deal, until I made s in Sichuan.

I often narrated that story during my public speeches, because it was also an education for others. The situation of street girls was neither relevant to morality nor sexuality. We could easily figure it out in another way, who should be accountable for these rural children? These children were citizens of this nation and had the right to work, but the government didn't provide them jobs. To fend for themselves, they had to go to the personnel market and were hired as nominal waitresses but actual street girls. What would you do if you were a teenager from a countryside who had never entered a big city before and didn't understand mandarin?

So, we should deliver our education towards the public about this field. However, that becomes less essential for more and more netizens begin to sympathize with these street girls.

(3) Objective conditions of sexual transmission

① There are ever fewer cases of abduction and coercion in prostitution.

I hadn't seen such a single case in Dongguan, Guangdong, though I was always told that girls were abducted and forced into prostitution. I said that I had met at least 200 street girls but no one was forced. Later I saw such cases in Sichuan, but the number was still rare.

Residents of Dongguan said: "At the beginning, the bosses were so silly that they wanted to lock up the girls as what was shown in movies. But it turned out to be impossible. Because Dongguan enjoyed the integration of urban and rural areas and was highly developed, the boss couldn't supervise a street girl round-the-clock. He should allow her to pee, right? And then she might be gone and became a salesgirl in the opposite store. The salary there was not so much less than before—maybe 20% lower. So, she could get other jobs and couldn't be locked up. The more prosperous the district is, the less likely there exists coercion. Even if she was confined, the other bosses would bail her out. It's called horizontal competition."

Later I found out that the abduction only occurred in remote places, such as Sichuan. First, the economy there was so bleak that the girls did not have a job. After being a street girl, she couldn't run away, or would suffer starving. Second, the local "sex industry" was so underdeveloped that she couldn't move to another entertainment place which didn't force girls, nor move to an upscale place. And there were no other bosses around to poach her. Besides that, the profit of prostitution was extremely low, the boss barely made much money, so they had to put street girls locked up.

I need to say more about that. Abduction and coercion are not the unique features of "sex industry". Those occur in many other industries, even in decent ones. Some people may turn amentia men into coal miners and some white-collar workers are forced to work overtime. The government cannot only be against prostitution and cannot focus on the punishment of street girls. Market economy should play its role in this issue to reduce abduction and coercion from root.

② What have the street girls suffered?

Some keep saying street girls are wretched victims of evil "sex industry" and are in great danger. Then they say in indignation: "Why do you support the legalization of street girls? Would you like your wife and daughter to lead such a perilous life?".

I agreed that at first, but later, in Shenzhen, my female postgraduate student lived door to door with three street girls who jointly hired a procuress. The procuress did many work, such as doing sentry-go and screening the guests and might be scolded if did anything wrong. My graduate student wrote her master's thesis based on that. After reading that thesis, I kept thinking the reason why these three little girls could do that. Then I got the answer—they are free people. So, if they were really legalized, they would have plenty of ways to protect themselves.

Mining can also cause death but mining is lawful for the workers are legal and free. Therefore, employers have to implement safety measures, scientists to identify new safer methods, and the state to protect workers' rights. As a result, although mining still cause death, yet no one say it is illegal.

③ Street girls don't earn much money.

If a street girl could go to Dongguan, Guangdong, it would not be the first time that she had gone far, and if she would be a street girl there, it also couldn't be the first time. The first karaoke lounge I went to in 1998 was in the middle range. The payment of street girls was not bad. It was about six or seven hundred yuan a night, at least 500–1,000 yuan. They dressed well and made up. At one sight of them, others would know they worked in a mid-range lounge. However, the lounge was small and kept only six or seven street girls, 10 at most. It was not big or splendid but good enough. Street girls could easily get 5,000 yuan or so a month there. At that time (1998) in Dongguan, that earnings could rival that of the workers of high class.

Basing on that, I carefully did some accounts for them in my first book, such as earnings of street girls and boss. The conclusion was that they could only earn a little bit more than the average wage of workers.

China leads the world in mathematics, but people at the bottom don't make accounts. Even most of the red-light district's bosses are, in fact, confused in this field. A beautiful top-billing street girl could attract many guests, so the boss gave her a pay rise. But then she left. The boss told me about that. What would you do if you were me? How could I tell him? He didn't understand the concept of cost accounting.

We always assume that people are rational, only harmed by economics. In fact, half Chinese at least are not economic or rational man, and in that case, 80% people are not. Being a street girl or running a hair salon are all gambling to them. The Chinese are born to gamble and don't account cost in that.

Street girls also dare to gambling. What did she know before she came to a red-light district? She knew nothing. Even if she had done prostitution before, she still did not know how many whoremasters were there. She had the courage to come, just because someone had said it was easy to earn money there. Without any authentic basis, she dared to go by herself. A little girl should be timid towards the evil world. But she was not and left for Dongguan alone. For us, if we were going to leave, we might consider the place where we could live, but she didn't even think about that. Most of girls coming for the first time were willing to accept work only for that could make more money. In fact, it did not earn that much. So why did they dare to make gambling? Because there's no other ways to go.

For most of the street girls, their kinsfolk knew what they were doing. Nowadays, the family running business together are becoming popular, because there is a family effect: the business that my relatives work in must be good, the salary must be high and the security can be guaranteed. It is hard for girls from village keeping relatives from knowing their jobs. But they try hard to keep that secret, such as by sending less money home. Sometimes they sent 600 yuan a month and sometimes 1,000 yuan. If their parents asked about her job, she would say it was a supermarket cashier. Parents didn't know the salary, so they told kid not to save so much but to enjoy nutritious food. Next time, they can only send 800 yuan.

But there were too many rural people working in towns. Without high income, they couldn't send back so much money. The only job that provided such high salary was being street girls. Because they didn't need to worry about food and accommodation which were generally provided by their boss. Though the condition might be not good, yet the salary was relatively higher than the average wage of workers. So, the extra was equivalent to their own savings.

④ Why do they do prostitution?

After being street girls for several months, many street girls are unable to take other jobs. Only a few can stay in lounge for half a year above, and if she is flexible enough, she can run a small business. Without sufficient capital in hand, she can help others do business or procurement to save money. For street girls over 30, they've done something else before, so if they stop working as a street girl, they can go back to jobs they did before. It is especially true for women with children, because they change the workplace frequently like doing part-time job. And they assume there is no difference between jobs. But for girls with only three years education (who always say they graduate from the junior high school but in fact haven't learnt anything at all), they will face that problems. Many street girls, especially the less educated and the young, are unable to do other jobs. If being street girl is her first job though that is very few, and she comes into this business under the delusion that she can earn more money, she would probably be trapped. After all, she earns 10–20 percent more than average workers. If she leaves, she will come back a few months later because she can notice the salary gap.

The main reason for being street girls is fellow villagers who are also the main reason for rural people leaving home for work. The current detaining education is to lock up the street girls arrested. Nominally, it is education, but in fact it is the punishment. Because only fellow villagers and relatives are functional in educating them. Street girls are willing to go with fellow villagers and relatives, even with less salary, because fellow villagers can give them hope. They think—"This fellow is reliable and leads a better life, so she may be the person who brings hope to get me out of this terrible place". That is common sense and human nature.

In Dongguan, even if there is only one guest two days, street girls can easily get 3,000 yuan a month which is not lower than others. In Beijing, if they can get about 5,000 yuan a month, that will be enough, but if just 3,000 yuan, the disparity will become obvious. However, relatives and fellow villagers will help her keep going. "Ant tribe" (Low-income and poor living groups in China) and "Beijing drifter" (People who are not from Beijing, but live and work in Beijing) are all caused by having no fellow villagers or relatives. If they had some, they wouldn't seem so pathetic. Look at sellers at the food market, they earn no less than you or even more than you. And they can become millionaires within five years. How do they get that? By fellows and relatives. We are Chinese, but scholars always regard ourselves as westerners and base researches on that to deal with problems. They always assume us as free people just like economists regard us as rational people. But actually, we are not. It was nonsense.

⑤ Poverty is not the only possible reason.

Whoremasters commonly ask 3 questions: "Where are you from?" The street girl usually answers with the name of a prefecture-level city or region; "How old are you"18—all street girls will say that; "How many people have you made sex with today?" None. It's always those three questions.

Then the girls will be asked the reason to be street girls. In the early years, the answer was miscellaneous. But now they say it is because of poverty, and poverty is the most acceptable reason.

After getting to know more, we began to talk about the situation about their family. Then I found that poverty was not the only reason for being street girls. A commissioner in a country is eligible enough to be included in upper class and definitely has sufficient money but his daughter was a street girl. There was also a sophomore working in a low-end hair salon during summer holidays. She was not suffering any difficulty at that time, but just wanted to do that. I would never believe it without seeing it with my own eyes. So, the so-called poverty is just a popular excuse, and all people can use it.

How poor is it on earth? Most street girls have brothers. At first, they didn't talk about that, but when I said I was a professor in a university, they would tell me their brother was studying in university, too. "How could your parents afford all the fees? They are needy farmers. Who support your brother's tuition and how much is it? Why do you know that and even the expenses for food and accommodation?" Then she told us she covered most of expense. Sometimes I said bluntly to my students present: "Maybe some of your sisters were doing this job to support you!".

In rural areas, boys are invaluable but girls are valueless, so it's common for parents to bring up boys at the cost of sacrificing the benefits of girls. This is not because of poverty but gender inequality.

Another reason is that there are patients in the family. Especially patients are their parents (No matter what disease it is), girls would be street girls because that could help them get more money to parents which is a way to show their filial piety. A girl in Guangxi insisted on dyeing her hair and didn't listen to her parents' advice. As a result, her scalp was burned and to restored it cost her parents a lot of money. Then she became a street girl to earn money because it's also filial to pay back parents' money.

Later, I found it was our outsider that conjectured the reason of being street girls. We consider there is a cliff, and one single mistake will cause eternal regret. To verify that, we went to the Northeast Region of China and asked the street girls there: "What did you do before?" Then we found that almost no one made prostitution as their first job. They had done some work before though that was not very decent. For example, they did serving at a restaurant or worked as a coolie in a hair salon. What they could do were just those jobs, and then gradually became street girls.

My female students chatted with street girls and were told: "In this street, the hair salons on this side are standard and even have no massage, while those on the other side are not only doing massage, but also having prostitution". My students asked her: "Did you work in that standard hair salon before?" She said: "Yes, the boss still knows me now, and sometimes I go to his salon to scrounge free meals." "Do you remember when you move from that standard salon to this one?" She replied:" I remember that day when my boss wanted to dismiss me. He said the business was slack and I should find another place for myself. Then I came here". That's exactly what she said. It seemed to her just a block away, and she didn't think there was a big difference between prostitution and hairdressing. Because all she did in both salons was being coolie. She was not a hair stylist and just helped fill the water bucket and swept the floor. But she might lead a little bit better life as a street girl.

"What do you want to do in the future?" "I would like to go home and run a small shop." All street girls would answer in that way and it seems that is their perpetual dream. However, a student of mine has kept in contact with two changers (who used to be street girls) by phone for more than two years, and no one really starts a shop. They still do some odd jobs and occasionally come back to be street girls.

Is it because of poverty? No. That is the result of social solidification, namely the vicious class inheritance. The bottom mass, especially women, who have no education background, can only stay in the bottom of society. The only way to change the situation is to marry a gentleman in the "upper class". From street girls' point of view, a gentleman is who runs a small business. Even if he is a salesman and goes out every day on a motorcycle, they would think they have someone to rely on, then they marry him. That is their destiny. From another perspective, let's take a look at the ordinary waitresses at the bottom of the service industry, what can they do other than street girls? Nothing. So, there is not such a deep gap between street girl and waitresses especially no moral reasons involving.

(4) The life connotation of sexual communication

4.1 Street girls' self-esteem

Once when I left a "red light district", a street girl, more than 30 years old, said: "you are eligible to marry me". Then several reporters and students asked me for my answer. Someone even relayed: A street girl wanted to marry me. Every time when I was asked about this question, I would reply: "The street girl's words moved me but your question hurts me."

"First of all, are you sure you really don't know what that means? Her words show that she treats me as a common person not a whoremaster and no longer regards me as a bad person. So, do I need to answer that question?"

"Then, does she really want to marry me? No. They just say I am a good man and good enough to marry her. Do you really think she want to marry up? No, it's just a compliment to me."

When I investigated in a red-light district, Go Home Often was a smash hit at that time. A young street girl said the lyrics were well-written. I said that was not because of lyrics itself but you who was deeply moved by that. In their community, they sat there dully and stiffly waiting for whoremasters. Then hearing that song, they must be extremely aggrieved. Such a song can be sung to the white-collar middle class, but it is completely a hurt to women workers at the bottom.

4.2 Street girls' pride

If a person didn't want to have sex with a street girl, that would be a huge humiliation to her. Firstly, she can't earn money and secondly, that behavior is called "Titai" which means a whoremaster choose a street girl but deem that she is no sexy. In their community, once that happened, they would fully lose face and have to leave. She might have been doing well here, earning enough money, but because of that she lost her job and confidence. So, street girls hate "Titai" most.

Sometimes, street girls don't need generous tips. Because the other street girls don't know that but know the "set fare" (money that guests give to the boss). The more the set fare is, the more the street girl values. And that will make her proud. We may think it is not worthwhile, but in such a small place, that little pride can bring her great happiness, for the life is too monotonous and dull. Actually, it's just human nature. Take an example, if you privately give a housing-sale lady 1000 yuan, of course she will be happy, but still not as happy as you buy a house from her. That is not about economics but about sociology.

4.3 Independence of street girls

Outsiders think street girls seem pathetic and are muddling along. But there is another side of her that isn't seen and known well.

Once I bluntly asked a street girl: "If you married and your husband discovered your experience, what will you do?" Guess what she said "Marry a chicken and share the coop, marry a dog and share the kennel. I make money by myself. If he wanted to break up, I would discard him first. Well, what an insular person he is."

There was a small group of street girls in Shandong, and one of them posted on the message wall that: the wife is plain boiled water and I am coke; but if I become a wife, I'll still be coke—I didn't remember well but that was the general idea.

Guangdong has been cracking down on pornography since 1980. Those who were street girls at that time are now 50 years old. Are they all not married? And do all of them have been divorced and come to a bad end?

At the beginning, once getting money, street girls would go to shopping to buy "street girl outfit" which was extremely tawdry and gaudy. However, they would dress themselves as ladies within three months. That is called the rapid adaption into the city life. Then they had some connections and began to select guests and knew about worldly wisdom which could help them become city dwellers. The living conditions might not be improved much, but at least they were independent.

I am a teacher at university and have seen many rural students becoming fashionable within a short time. That is the same reason. The point is whether you give her a chance, and whatever it is, it will be better than staying in the countryside. Otherwise, why did the educated youth want to head back to the cities? (After the founding of PRC, to address the employment problem, some educated youth were assigned to rural areas. In 1977, Gaokao resumed, the educated youth did everything possible to come back to city, even physically harmed themselves.)

4.4 The new generation of street girls

In the summer of 2010, there was a nationwide campaign against pornography. We went out to investigate whether the campaign was effective but were shocked by new findings.

Stepping into the street girls' rest room in a high-end karaoke lounge, I saw a large sheet of red paper posted on the wall and words in it were disciplines street girls followed: do not ignore guests, do not grab guests' microphone, do not drink guests' beverages. And the most unbelievable one is to do not beat or scold the guest! What disciplines they were. Then I was informed these young girls were all in post-90s generation. They claimed to be street girls, but only entertained each other not guests. If a guest only invited one street girl, the rest would come along even without pay and after drinking too much, they would become crazy. The guest complained and the manager entreated street girls not to do that again. But it didn't work. Because they those street girls thought they were beautiful and sexy and if the manager dismissed them, they could find an even better lounge. The manager said sadly: "They don't want to make money. They just come for fun. And I have to provide them food and accommodation and give them money. How stupid I am."

That is called ever-changing life. My old idea about street girl is out of date and should be updated. Professor He (Chunrui He) in Taiwan has noticed that phenomenon long before and has written several books about it, called "bold ladies". Therefore, it is not enough to focus on "poverty theory" and we should also consider the independent choice of women. And some coinages are supposed to be popularized, such as female body autonomy and erotic autonomy.

Surely, that case is an individual one. But if I had to conclude one reason, that would be my fault. I am unable to take all factors into consideration and record 100 or 200 kinds of cases. Even if I can, someone would ask me: "Which one is most important?" How could I answer that? So, when it comes to the cause of prostitution, it can't purely attribute to poverty or the moral corruption. Because the reason is diverse and beyond our imagination.

4.5 How many street girls are there in China?

Nowadays, people always overestimate the number of street girls. Some say it is 10 million and even 20 million. Now we need to make it clear. Whoever says it, or asks me for it, I will raise three questions in return.

Firstly, "What is your definition of street girls"? International feminism counts stripteasers in it, do you? Do mistresses count? They also trade sex for money. Now some people actually count all the women working in entertainment places, including hair salons. Some even didn't have any and made the estimation groundlessly.

Secondly, "Which kind of girls can be defined as street girls?" Does it include those who do massage, offer escort service or help guests do hand job (masturbation), but not have sex with guests? Without these perceptions, one just blurts out 20 million, isn't that just for fun?

And thirdly, let's do some elementary arithmetic. If each street girl receives a lot of guests per day, the number of street girls should inversely reduce. In Beijing, if a street girl received 20 guest a day, 1000 street girls would be enough and the redundant would have no business. But some people on the one hand assert street girls receive many guest, and on the other hand say there are many street girls, dare you inform your elementary teacher of that?

We overestimate street girls' income due to our overestimation of the number of guests they receive. Remember: without buying, selling cannot exists. When I went to Dongguan for the first time, I stared at six hair salons from 3 p.m. to 12 p.m. to figure out the number of street girls, of men coming in and out, of those who were accompanied by street girls and of motorcycles which were parked there to solicit guests. I counted all the men including those who only had a look, and wrote numbers down. After my calculation, I found that it averagely took two days for a street girl to receive one guest.

Professor Liao and Wu, both senior scholars, led a survey which showed it took 1.5–2 days to get a guest—not as much as ordinary people think. It is also said that some street girls make a good fortune, having a house and a car. Yes, that might be true, but the chance is extremely small, 1% or so, which can be negligible.

Only the growing number of guests could cause the increasing number of street girls. In recent years, however, the population of street girls is mounting but guests are not, leading to the descending average guest reception and more intensified competition for guests. As a result, relative poverty among street girls emerges. Now the market is in the recession all over the country. Street girls who used to work in karaoke lounge or splendid club now are working at hair salon or bath house. They have no other way to go in this slack market. Look at the people soliciting guests on the street, some of them look like models. Under such circumstances where the total number of the sex trade has not changed, the number of street girls is meaningless and what is significant now is the relative poverty of them.

So, conservatively speaking, the street girls in China who really provide sex service are just over 1 million, or 3 million at most. That is exactly got by calculation, not by estimation, because we have made a nationwide survey and knew how many men make sex with street girls and the average guests a street girl receiving per day. With those, we can have the results. If you don't believe me, please give us a more convincing method.

On the surface, people complain about the large number of street girls, but in fact some criticize the gap between the rich and the poor: street girls earn so much, but I just get that little. Some scold the corruption, or even blatantly blame reform and opening up. So, be careful when you curse street girls, because others may ask you: "You say no one is willing to join prostitution, but why are there so many street girls? Who forced them to do it? What do you remind us of? And when you say that street girls are rich, don't you mean that is the way to become rich?".

There's a paradox here. If a street girl is arrested and fined but has no money for all her money is sent home or given her boyfriend, she can only borrow money from boss. Then, she will become a slave suffering oppression and exploitation and has to make efforts to earn money to pay off debts. Conversely, even if she has money, what will happen after being fined? Quit? No. She has to redouble her efforts to recover the loss.

Instead of being caught and fined, what street girls frighten most is to notify their family. When a street girl is caught, police have to inform her relatives, for one cannot just evaporate without any news. But once it happens to street girls, the good intention will become the most terrible punishment. Because gossips can spread rapidly in a rural area, and that notification will be a humiliation to her family forever.

(5) The possibility of sexual transmission
5.1 The degree of importance in AIDS in street girls' lives.

After participating in AIDS prevention work, I found experts on AIDS prevention are very active and work hard, but they always focus on a superficial facet—street girls. Almost all of us have seen street girls because they can be easily found in some kinds of streets or hair salons. Unfortunately, most of us only regard them as street girls, ignoring that they are real people who have boyfriends, husbands or lovers and emotions. They need someone to share feelings with and depend on. But how does AIDS come about? Some country girls became street girls at 13. Does the AIDS come from them? No, it is from men and they transmit it to street girls. However, now, street girls are criticized as the source of AIDS. Don't you think that is against the common sense and the conscience?

The experts believe that AIDS are spread by street girls and direct them to "put on the condom" but those are extremely unreasonable. Then I told them: "You have better professional knowledge than us, but lack common sense and conscience because you regard them as patients not the real people. If not, why don't you ever ask them about their children and their boyfriends, husbands or lovers? Knowing nothing but you don't ask about. That shows you don't care it at all. Do you know how much money she makes, what does she spend her money on? No, you don't know."

I told the experts, from the perspective of street girls, the most significance is to make money and the second is to be safe. However, the so-called safety is not relevant to AIDS but avoid being beaten, killed, robbed, stolen, burned, etc., that is, avoid being bullied by guests. And the third is pregnancy and gynaecological disease. I said: "You are female, why do you need a man to inform you of that? They have sex every day, so they must be afraid of being pregnant. Getting Venereal disease (VD) has some symptoms which can be seen by others. Once getting that, they will be despised and knocked out. As a result, they cannot continue to work and get no money. However, AIDS has no visible symptom, they don't need to worry about it."

"What's more, street girls who are married and have children have to consider children' schooling and parenting and what to do if their husbands left them. The last is AIDS. They asked: 'Once getting AIDS, I will die immediately, right?' I replied: 'No, there's an incubation period.' 'How long is it?' 'Two or three years.' 'Oh, that is not a big problem. I may die at any time. Don't worry about that.' So, as I said, this kind of AIDS prevention program purely cannot hit the point, because for you, AIDS prevention is the first goal, but for them, that ranked fourth or even fifth."

Actually, street girls, especially the unmarried, are most afraid of abortion which terrifies girls all over the world especially here in China. Because after abortion, they may get half dead. One street girl goes to hospital accompanying by three others, and when they come back, the boss will know the consequence, saying: "If you want to leave, then go, and I will hire some new girls." That "blooding baby" is put on a small tray in front of them. Seeing that, are they still willing to be street girls? No. And no matter how rich and powerful you are and how excellent your husband is, one cannot evade having babies. There are few Chinese women who dare to say that they will not have children, except these who have received high education. Abortion can smash one's confidence, and the boss knows that better than us.

The intellectuals, around 40 years old, always tackle things with theories and regard the average income as the standard line. That is nonsense. Dose the same amount of money deliver the same meaning to different people? For Bill Gates, he can easily get 1 million, but what about for people from the bottom? In several "red light districts", street girls have no condom just because condoms are expensive. "Expensive?", others were astounded: "It just costs two yuan!" I replied: "Even if it was fifty cents, they would still think it is expensive. Because they have no spare money to buy it."

Some scholars asked: "Every time when we distribute free condoms, street girls always snatch them, but they don't use." I said: "She cannot use up all and can sell the extra with the price of 1 yuan to others. In some places, 100,000 condoms can be distributed within a month at a small 'red light district', then street girls can sell them even to 20 km away. Do you know that?" Well, they are all medical professionals, so it cannot blame them if they don't know that.

In fact, this topic always frets me. Can street girls decide whether to wear a condom or not? Even the whoremaster's wife cannot decide it. The experts don't make efforts to educate whoremasters but aim at street girls, doesn't that come out of contempt? In Amsterdam, street girls hire "condom police", and if a whoremaster is unwilling to wear condom, a group of people will besiege him and educate him and even continue to follow him after he left. Then he will remember to wear a condom next time.

5.2 Sexual transmission—first between street girls and her boyfriends

What's the Chinese women need most? Inner sustenance. The capacity of supporting family is just at the second place. The man they choose must be their inner sustenance. Now you may understand their relationship with pimps, or procures or bosses. A 17-year-old street girl called her boyfriend and said coquettishly, "Oh dear, you just need to lie to me that you love me. That will be enough. Okay?" After a while, she said: "I know you take my money to find other street girls. But it does not matter, because you love me and that is enough. I know you are taking drugs. That is not a big problem and I will still give you my money." She just wanted love and to hear "I love you". Then she would give all her hard-earned money to the pimp or so-called boyfriend.

These pimps deliberately look for street girls to be their girlfriends and then scrounge for money from them. What's worse, pimps generally have more than two girlfriends and live off all of them.

I had been in a place for few days, and then the boss, in his 40s, noticed I was so sympathetic to street girls and wanted to give them money. Then he lectured me: "Even if you gave them your total fortune, it would make no difference because they would immediately give that money to their pimps." Economically, pimps are the people who control and exploit street girls. But they are also street girls' boyfriends. That's the combined one. Just with money, one can only manage street girls but cannot control them, and is unable to stop them from leaving. However, with love, one can take physical control over them, especially for who has a honey mouth. Now you may understand why so many college students are induced by rural migrant workers, some even for years. "Love" is the pivotal reason!

In Inner Mongolia, my male student visited a pimp who had seven street girls. That could be called a big business. And we asked how he achieved that. He just said something else and didn't answer the question. After a while, he brought a street girl and my students asked me to have a look. Then I noticed her eyes were filled with love towards the pimp. That is love control.

And then I asked myself: "is that strange?" No, that can happen in any woman. It's not a peculiarly street girls' problem but a general cultural issue.

But after experiencing more, I changed my view towards pimps. In 2010, I came back to a red-light district and found there were more and more mom-and-pop stores. Not all of them were real couples, and they just lived together, did business together, but enjoyed deep affection. I met several pairs in Tianjin, Shandong and Guangxi and had nice chats with them. Huang Yingying criticized me: "You keep saying the word 'pimp', because you only regard them as pimps. Now you just like what I used to be. At that time, I had a strong prejudice against online dating and didn't believe the online love could have a happy ending. But now, my niece is married to a man she knows through internet. At the thought of that, I always feel guilty to her."

5.3 The bottleneck of prevention education is not ignorance, but the blind mobility.

The common sense of AIDS transmission shows that the less the mobility of high-risk groups have, the more it is conducive to transmission prevention. However, street girls are in high mobility. Street girls who work in the same place for more than three months are very few. Most of them stop in one place for a month, then move to thousands of kilometers away, like from Heilongjiang to Hainan, from Hainan to Sichuan. That is true not only for street girls who work in high-level hotel, but also for those in the low hair salons. The young and undereducated street girls from the bottom live in a closed environment and lack life experience. So, once a half-true message is sent to them, they will go to thousands of kilometers away alone. As long as there is a person she knows—even if she only knows the name, she will dare to go. It's not because she is bold but because she has no other information and ways. Where can she go if business is bleak here? How does she know where the "red light district" is? How does she know where business is great? It totally depends on blind guessing. Other street girls or relatives talk about something by phone and she accidentally hears that, thinking the business seems good there, then she leaves. That is their way of survival and they have no other choices.

If a street girl stays in the same place for a month, she will hardly get more guests, because guests like new street girls. Some whoremasters, even on their first visit to a strange lounge, can tell how long street girls have worked. We did a simple survey in street girls' workplaces and found that almost every street girl will say: "I just came here today." They won't say: "I have been here for more than a month", or they will have no guests. Therefore, they have to move frequently but that helps AIDS transmission. When investigating in red-light districts, I was told more than once: "A street girl who worked here before had venereal disease (VD) and took drugs". Then I asked when she left and where she went, but they didn't know. Given these circumstances, how can we conduct our education? Besides that, the current campaign against pornography also forces them to change places. So, do you think street girls will voluntarily participate in HIV prevention?

5.4 Street girls are genuine experts in transmission prevention.

Nowadays, many people in China who work to prevent AIDS do make great efforts and come into contact with some street girls. But their biggest deficiency is that they always postulate street girls know nothing about disease prevention. However, many street girls have worked for two to three years and receive the average of 200–300 whoremasters. Are they really not afraid of death? No. They have developed a lot of effective methods to prevent disease, but you don't know that.

In Dongguan, a street girl told me a shed next to a karaoke lounge did prostitution and had blue movies (The shed was in middle level and had good conditions). All the movies she showed were selected and about foreigners who wore condom. She would show movies to guests. If guests didn't want to wear it, she would say: "Look, foreigners also wear condoms." Whoremasters took a look—oh, it is really—then put on it.

I didn't know that before, and I would never think of that if she hadn't told me.

How to prevent AIDS? Now, condoms are the evidence of prostitution, but if you find condoms, you should extenuate their crime, because wearing condoms is conducive to AIDS prevention. Given that point, one needn't to do much educational intervention. When I said that at the National AIDS Prevention Conference in 2000, everyone nodded and agreed. But until now it hasn't been widely recognized.

(6) The other part of sexual transmission: male guests (which mean whoremasters)
6.1 What do male guests buy?

I have contacted a lot street girls, but it is difficult to meet some male guests, because they just leave away as soon as getting satisfied. I've talked with a few guests. Some aged ones don't leave immediately, and they sit there, talking with others. Or, they chat for several hours before entering the street girl's room. I like to talk with such kind of people. But for the rest, I have to sit down and lead a formal interview.

At a karaoke lounge in Kunming, Yunnan, I asked some guests for a light, then drank wine and chatted with them. To show their generosity, they treated me to drinks. Chatting for a while, I was asked: "Come for fun?" I knew that was the time to deliver our purpose, then replied: "We are from the Renmin University of China and come to do a research." But three quarters of guests said: "Sorry. I won't join in that" "It has nothing to do with me" ... the talk had to be stopped.

Finally, I found a procuress as the intermediary. She certainly had a good memory, or she could not work for a long time. She was able to remember men who ever asked price, let alone other guests. The procuress knew men very well and was considerate enough, so it was easy for her to get acquainted with these guests. Her referral represented the advancement to success. In total, she introduced nine groups to me and each had 3 to 6 people.

Later, I had some person-to-person talk in Ya'an and Luzhou and at Tricycle Drivers Association, where had more whoremasters from the bottom. They didn't care and were not afraid of much and admitted that they were whoremaster. But they didn't tell me some deeper things. Indeed, such formal s easily made people nervous, no matter who they were. The only way to solve the problem is to drink wines, but drinking is not a strength in our team. I am often laughed at for that: "How can you do research with that little drinking capacity?". I reply: "But I have to do research anyway."

Then I wrote some articles on whoremasters. It was not about research, just some of my discoveries and understandings. For example, why does a man exist who cannot satisfy his wife living with him but goes out to find street girls? When I give speeches to women, I always say, "If you cannot figure that out, I will doubt whether you are married or not."

What do whoremasters look for from street girls? One is to look for gorgeous women. A female student asked me: "What kind of women are gorgeous to whoremasters?" I replied: "Coquettish". Because in the general situation and occasions, one cannot find a coquettish woman, but money can find such one. Second is for service. Whoremasters can ask street girls to do anything he wants and doesn't need to scruple to her feelings, but they cannot do that to their wives or girlfriends, or they may break up. Third is for intimacy. How escort girls make money? Through company and sweet tongues, and by that whoremaster will be willing to give money. If they want to have sex, please give the extra money.

And the last is for sexual skills. But we need to make it clear that not all street girls can do it. It is said that there is a "SEX ISO" in Dongguan, but it is not true. Believe it or not, many "ISO" on the Internet are written by pimps themselves, which are actually for advertising. But as the story spread, I was asked to talk about such skills in my elite women's class. I wondered and asked them: "Do you want to satisfy yourselves, or to hold your husbands' hearts? If you want to hold their hearts, it will be in vain because wife can never rival the street girl in this aspect. Because the two are different in identity. You aren't willing to be regarded as goods and you believe in reciprocal love. But street girls are not, they can be treated as toys. So, a woman can be a wife, but a wife may not be a 'woman' ".

So, if a man has sex with street girls, there is only one reason: they believe sex, love and marriage are different items which can be separated—even for a while. There is a "public toilet theory" among men: "I don't love her (street girls) and don't want to marry her. It is just like I want to pee while in the street and find a place to solve it. So, what are you (wife) worried about?" Surely, the wife won't believe but can't outargue him, so they have to say: "Ok, fine. I will do what you have done". However, would they really do that? So, the question is: Can the female control and drive their lust independently?

Street girls share the same idea with whoremasters and regard them as wallets. As a result, they are independent. A street girl in Lanzhou was killed and 1,100 love letters were found under her bed which were all written in the same year to her husband, the legal husband. Could you say she had no love and no marriage? No. She just separated sex from love in order to earn money to raise children. Besides, is prostitution out of her own lust? Does she expect that? No, that is to satisfy a guest's lust. She's just renting out her genital organ.

There are few research about men and I also don't know men well. Anyway, when they talk about having sex, it always carries many other implications. When my students and I interviewed some male guests, we asked: "What can be called go-whoring exactly? What is different between having sex with street girls and with wife?" The answers were assorted but some people couldn't even say a word. The writer calls it "thinking with the lower body". I'm not that lofty, and I think it's because our education of sociology of sex doesn't perform well. They have to learn some words and concepts before they can answer the question. So, we can't blame anyone for what should be figured out by ourselves.

Our biggest misunderstanding is that we always think the police only catch street girls but not whoremasters. Actually, that varies in different situations. We all know the term "revenue generation" (use one's own favourable conditions for the unit to increase income), so who helps increase more money? Street girls earn little, and even if you killed them, they still couldn't pay a lot. But what about whoremasters? Even though they claim having no money, they certainly have a boss, a wife or a mother. Anyway, there is definitely a person they afraid of, so they have to obediently pay money! If you don't believe that, please check the report of Public Security Bureau, and you will find out there are more whoremasters than street girls in the list.

6.2 What is the relationship between whoremasters and street girls?

In my previous books, I involuntarily assumed male guests and street girls were antagonistic. But now with accumulated experiences, I realize the reality is far more complicated. In Sichuan, I witnessed a soldier who was going to take a street girl home and married her. The street girls around them were touched to cry, but it seemed not a big deal for the street girl who was going to get married. After all, she had been dating the soldier for at least a year.

But then I pondered: was it still called go-whoring? Was she still a street girl? So, later I wrote a short article: Who is street girl? She is a street girl under particular situation and time and when she goes shopping, she is a customer; when she comes home, she is the wife and daughter, and the mother of her kids. Street girl is just a role that she plays. Various roles are comprised one's identity. So why dose "street girl" become their most predominant label? Now we can see ever more street girls are actually part-time and amateurish, and prostitution becomes a temporary and one-off job. And they serve as street girls by chance when they go out or travel. Who could be a lifetime street girl? No one. So, if you don't know that, please shut up.

So, I object to the notion of "lostgirl". Indeed, that sounds much more pleasant than "whore". But it can only be addressed within the particular period and event. For example, it's immoral to spit everywhere and if you do that, I will call you a "lostman". Will you be angry about that? However, if I called you "lostman" all the time basing on that little incidental, you would be undoubtedly indignant about that.

Go-whoring is also a kind of interpersonal relationship but related to money. And it is similar to other male-female relationships which include fight, love, or unrequited love. But many of us look down upon street girls and whoremasters and regards them as shameless people—academically, that is called "stigmatization." In fact, many street girls are rescued by the whoremasters, at least we have seen that in Sichuan. Bold guests made phone calls to the police station and reported there were some girls being abducted. Then the police came to the bar, just standing there without saying a word, the boss would be frightened and said: "Do you want to leave? Then, just go." The guests who were not bold enough would phone street girls' parents, saying: "Your daughter is ill and now she is in…" Once the boss answered the phone from street girls' parents, he would allow street girls to leave. He said: "I'm a business man, not a murderer. I won't try to make trouble."

6.3 "My lover is a street girl"

When I interview male guests, I always ask questions involving wife and lover to make a contrast. Once, I chatted about lover with a driver of the three-wheel motor.

He talked about that for a long time, but finally sighed: "Alas, without paying her money, she is still not happy." I consoled him by saying that he ought to give some money. Then he said: "But there is no concession in the price." I was confused by his words and pled him to tell me the whole story. Then I was informed that his lover was a street girl and he knew her in a hair salon and had sex there. "But how can you call her your lover? She is a street girl." He replied: "She cooks dinner for me." Ok, fine. I failed.

I'm really stupid, you know. Street girls even do not cook for themselves but cook for whoremasters. It is the "true love". That whoremaster didn't lie to me. It was I who forgot the human nature. Of course, I can say he has so few requirements that is easy to be ingratiated, but does love have to be extremely romantic? I could have told him that: "She does that only for your money." But, what I want to know is the real him and he thought street girl was his lover. That's the fact. I have to embrace that. And the analysis relating it should be left for other researches.

Then I found that I held an oversimplified view about street girls and whoremasters. Anyway, I was too naïve.

6.4 Change in attitudes of male guests

In the last decade, men's attitudes towards street girls have been changed. When we went to a red-light district 10 years ago, it was still full of abuse towards street girls even from men who went whoring: "They are reduced to prostitution purely because of laziness." A great number of men have told me: "They can earn 1,000 yuan each month working in a factory, and can only earn 2,000 yuan being a street girl. There is not a big difference. So, why don't they work in a factory?".

I said: "Why don't you call it a doubling? If you are deducted half from your income, what will you do?".

At first, they didn't buy what I said and argued: "It is much easy for street girls to earn money, and they even needn't to exert any physical efforts." I said: "Is that really easy? Does that really not involve physical efforts? You go there every day and should know more than others. They sit there dully waiting for guests and at the meantime, suffering the troubles from the family. 'Your brother is ill, send money home.' 'I (Dad) want money, send me some.' The big bosses like you should experience more this kind of mental pressure than us. You have a company, so you have to deal with issues involving tax, debts and wastes. Street girls also experience those annoying problems, so why can't you understand them?".

What I said embarrassed them, and they said: "In that way, I do know more than you." I said: "Of course you know more than me. But, because you don't regard them as common people, and you don't think in that way."

My friend, the president of a hospital (mentioned before), have many buddies from Taiwan, China and Hong Kong, China. Some are Japanese technicians and local small-business owners. They all can be called people from high-society circles. When I talked about street girls to them, they said, "I can understand that. Those girls need money, and I have a surplus of money, so I will give them."

About in the last 5 years, the online public opinion has changed. If one sends a post scorning street girls, all replies will condemn the poster. Why? It is not because all people have some affairs with street girls, but that people ever more understand the meaning of "forced by life." Migrant workers, white-collar workers and all kinds of other people are suffering great life pressure. A catchword goes like that: "It is easy to come to this world but it not easy to stay alive in this world. And it is much more difficult to live in this world." Street girls share same feelings. On the other hand, the poster stands on the moral high ground and genteelly criticize street girls--no wonder others condemn him or her.

6.5 AIDS prevention among male guests

I must emphasize again: prostitution comes after go-whoring, so the AIDS transmission mostly attributes to 1whoremasters. But intervention programs designed today rarely aim at them. Of course, it is objectively difficult to guide whoremasters, because they would leave as soon as they finished and we cannot track them, while street girls are confined in their workplace. However, if we do not carry out AIDS prevention education to the male guests, all the previous efforts targeting street girls will be in vain. At red-light districts in Amsterdam, there is a good idea that we can learn from. Although there is no police officer arresting people involving prostitution and go-whoring, yet condom police are available. If a guest doesn't use a condom, condom police will begin their work as I said before.

However, we still have other measures to make s and intervention towards guests. In the relatively transparent "red-light districts", a substantial portion of guests will stay there for a while and we can avail that to begin our intervention and. Once I took six female graduate students to a "red light district" to make s. In all, they interviewed more than 70 whoremasters, with a rejection rate of about 50 percent, and 38 received their interview. But for me, the failure rate was close to 80%. It seems that this kind of research is more appropriate for women.

If a man interviews another man, the big problem will be: how to detect whether he tells lies or not and whether he brags or not. Among whoremasters who received my interview, they were either having-sex-many-times-a-day, or earning-money-by-go-whoring (They didn't need to pay street girls and street girls give money to them out of love). They were so "heroic". However, in red-light districts, I have seen with my own eye that many whoremasters were caught by police, cheated and extorted by others and taunted by street girls for impotence. Why can't I interview such a man? So, I have no way of telling fiction from fact. And actually, some plots in Strange Stories from a Chinese Studio also show the sexual myth in men's mind, which is a typical bias towards male. In this matter, I have no good idea to change people's cognition till now.

(7) I know about your life and you enrich my mind.

Every time when I give lessons to my students, I always ask a question: What is the biggest risk in doing publicity and education in red-light districts? Answers of them are "being extorted", "being defrauded", or "being induced to join them". Even some of my colleagues said: "Hi, Lao Pan, take me there and I swear I won't be disturbed."

I said: "Oh, you exposed. NOT QULIFIED. Why do you think they will disturb you? Are they demons or evils who want to harm you? You take them as foxtrels, but why don't you regard them as poor little girls or the equal people with you?".

Only once, there was a man who looked like in his thirties answering in the right way. He was a medical student and he said: "The biggest risk is the street girl may fall in love with you". Why? Because of your age, status, and the way you treat her. Other men look down at them and seemingly condescend to talk with them. But you sit down to talk with them in an equal manner and take her as the focus. Since her father or elder brother may not have treated her in the same way, she is certainly moved by that.

She falls in love with you. You can be grateful but have no way to respond her. And she maybe gets hurt by it. That is the biggest risk.

Once, purely out of curiosity and not of any, a female teacher insisted on having a small chat with a street girl. She asked me what question she should ask first. I said: "Talk something about her kids." She didn't believe that and said: "She is so young. How could she have kids?" I replied: "Just do it. As long as she hears that, her tears will come down" But she was even more incredulous. However, as a result, she and the young street girl huddled together and both wept.

Those questions are not related to knowledge but to the philosophy of life. A male doctor engaging in AIDS prevention said: "Mr. Pan, at the beginning, I didn't believe what you write, but now, after seeing you, I believe it." I said: "What do you mean? Do you think I look like a whoremaster?" He replied: "No. Just because you are affable."

That does not solely depend on affability. The sincerity and honesty are also indispensable in interpersonal communications. Once stepping into the bar, I cannot have much privacy. When I was in Dongguan, a procuress who helped me during my called my wife to have a small chat. It was so expensive to make long-distance calls at that time. And she called three times, each time lasting for more than half an hour. My wife told to her: "Let's hang up and I'll call you." However, the procuress didn't listen to that. Then I left, and so did she, but she still remembered to call me and told me she was going to leave.

After my first trip to the red-light district, I came home and wrote a book called What is Real and What is Absurd: An onto China's Underground Sex Industry. The title was conceived by my student. But, now, I notice that book carries strong stereotyped images. One is it only expresses the pathos of street girls but ignores their independent choice: for them, being street girls indeed is not the only option but it is a good one. Second is it improperly builds oppositions between guests and street girls and between street girls and bosses. Because I am brought up in the situation where was filled with the class struggles, so it's easy for me to discover those binary oppositions. That is completely unconsciously.

And then I decided to focus on the red-light district to figure out the way it works--that is the real sociology. But doing that for a long time, I find the way the red-light district works is not much different from other common commercial areas. We have investigated all the local people who have contact with the street girls. Academically, they are called "associated people" which include owners of newsstand, delivery men, drug sellers, doormen, and even the common residents. All I did was to figure out their relationship with "red light district". As a result, apart from red-light districts in development zones in Sichuan, others are just like common commercial districts and will become bleak once undergoing the anti-pornography campaign. There is really no great difference.

I always tell my students this: "After more than ten years' research, I find there is nothing to explore. The more research I conduct, the more I realize that street girls are just common people and not different from others. Actually, it is not there is really no difference, but the difference is not that obvious as we expect."

Once in Guizhou province, I walked for 16 km along the mountain road alone and felt exhausted. Some girls shouldering food, mineral water, instant noodles, and so on, covered themselves up though they were soaked with sweat, to avoid being tanned. The goods they carried weighted about 50 kg but they only earned two yuan. Street girls sitting next to them could earn 30 yuan each time. Then I thought, what's the difference? Why don't those girls do prostitution? I don't know. With extreme curiosity, I began my research.

I think all researchers who begin their research with this idea: Street girls are special! But gradually, I find that my research becomes: there is a class of "workers" who are not so different from other workers. But they are specially treated and scolded as "bad women" purely due to their work involving sex. So, is sex inherently bad, or is there something else that makes it so bad? If sex isn't so bad, and neither is money, then why do two things become bad when they are combined together? Don't tell me about so-called morality. How can you force others to obey your morality?

After all, the issue concerning money has been discussed a lot in China, but the sex issue is still not under discussion. Why is sex so precious and private and issues involving it so sensitive? Why does sex carry so many implications which cannot be used casually? Everyone has their own perspective and can express their opinions, but the community of sociology of sex has to answer those questions. As for me, I will work hard and keep fighting.

The manufacturer's authorised representative in the EU is Springer Nature Customer Service Centre GmbH, Europaplatz 3, 69115 Heidelberg, Germany. If you have any concerns regarding our products, please contact ProductSafety@springernature.com

Printed and bound by CPI Group (UK) Ltd, Croydon, CR0 4YY
30/09/2026
02225290-0007